A Green Witch's
Formulary

Deborah J. Martin

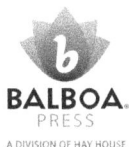

BALBOA.
PRESS
A DIVISION OF HAY HOUSE

ISBN: 978-1-4525-3709-2 (sc)
ISBN: 978-1-4525-3710-8 (e)

Library of Congress Control Number: 2011935116

Balboa Press books may be ordered through booksellers or by contacting:
    Balboa Press
    A Division of Hay House
    1663 Liberty Drive
    Bloomington, IN 47403
    www.balboapress.com
    1-(877) 407-4847

Printed in the United States of America

Balboa Press rev. date: 8/1/2011

For my husband, Pete: without his love and support, I would never have made it to where I am today. And for my spirit guides who gave me encouragement – and a kick in the pants when I needed it.

Table of Contents

Preface

The use of plants as both medicine and magical helpers goes back to the beginnings of Man. The earliest written records we have available to us date from the ancient Chinese and Babylonians about 5,000 years ago. Even as late as 1,000 years ago, people were combining their knowledge of the medicinal uses of plants with vocal spells for healing and other needs.

At some point in our more recent history, science took over and separated the plants' medicinal uses from their magical attributes. It was a gradual development, starting with Paracelsus and his alchemy (a forerunner to chemistry) in the 1500's. By the 1780's, scientists had learned to extract the individual chemicals from plants. The mid-1800's saw the first synthesis of organic compounds, and the rise of the use of chemicals instead of plants to treat illness. It wasn't until after World War I, however, that synthetic drugs truly began to replace organics to help Man. I, like many of my friends, prefer to combine what we now know scientifically with the more occult aspects of my green friends.

To solve a problem, I turned from book to book, trying to find an herbal solution. My research took me from scientific knowledge to ancient ways and back again. Along the way I've compiled favorites along with some helpful suggestions that I'd like to share with you. As always, please do your research first to ensure you won't be using herbs to which you may be allergic, or which causes an unfavorable interaction with other herbs and/or prescription medication.

As you research, you're going to come across terms that describe the therapeutic actions of herbs, and I've used some of them. These terms describe how an herb works on your body. For example, a *vermifuge* expels worms from the body while a *vermicide* kills worms. It's important to choose the correct action for a particular problem. You'll find a list describing the most widely used terms in the appendices.

Always remember that any herb you use in a magical application is going to interact with your body. Generally speaking, there are many herbs that provide the same effect, so you should be able to avoid allergens. If you feel you *must* use a poisonous herb or one to which you are allergic, handle it with gloves; definitely don't ingest it and, if you burn it, do not inhale the smoke.

Acknowledgments

This book would not be possible without the help of so many: first and foremost, the teachers at American College of Healthcare Sciences. To the hundreds who, over the centuries, have shared their knowledge in print and now electronically, both medicinal and magical: my profound thanks. To my friends at TW: you have helped shape this book in more ways than you can imagine. I love you all.

Medicinal

The medicinal dosages given within are for adults. Herbs should never be given to an infant less than six months of age unless under the care of a medical practitioner. As a general rule of thumb, other dosages are:

6-12 months	1/10 adult dose
1-5 years	¼ adult dose
6-12 years	½ adult dose
Over 70 years	¾ adult dose

Be sure the herb is safe to use not only for you, but for children, elderly, or frail persons. Some herbs are not safe to be used when pregnant or nursing, as whatever you take will make its way into your baby's body. Certain herbs have what is known as a low therapeutic margin. This means the correct dose can help, anything over that can harm or even kill.

As you research herbs and come up with your own recipes, you may want to combine herbs with different actions to achieve the desired results. For example, if you've got bronchitis and want to get rid of mucus in your lungs, you may want a demulcent to break up the mucus and an expectorant to get it all out. Or, if you are constipated, some herbs are very strong and can be irritating. Therefore, you'd combine a cathartic herb with a corrective and demulcent herb.

Don't expect overnight results. Illness (or dis-ease) is an imbalance in your body somewhere. Herbs work *with* your body to bring it back into balance. This takes a bit of time, so for a major or chronic problem, give a treatment at least ten days (and preferably thirty) before giving up and going on to something else. Remember: your body is unique to you. What works for me may not work for you and vice versa. It may take some experimentation to come up with a personalized solution.

If you're uncertain of *anything* herbal, please consult a qualified herbalist or naturopathic physician.

Acne

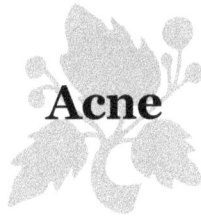

Acne is more than a teenager's problem—many older adults also have acne. It can be caused by a number of items: changes in hormone levels, allergies, and pollution, to name a few.

One of the first things you need to do is ensure that your acne isn't due to an allergy. You can ask your physician to perform allergy tests, or do an elimination diet. Eliminate "known offenders" (chocolate, eggs, sugar, peanut butter and processed cheese are the most common) from your diet for 2 weeks. Re-introduce them one at a time to see if there are any changes in your skin. If you discover an offender, eliminate it from your diet for at least a year.

Lifestyle Modifications

Start dry skin brushing before showering or bathing. To do this, purchase a natural bristle brush, preferably one with a long handle so you can reach all parts of your body. Prior to getting wet, brush your entire body with small, circular strokes, starting at the soles of your feet and working up your legs; from the palms of your hands to your shoulders; then at your neck, working down. In other words, always work towards the heart. Avoid your face, nipples and other "sensitive" areas: this brush is too harsh. It should take you around five minutes. This will help slough off dead skin cells, and stimulate the capillaries just under the surface as well as the lymph system, helping the skin do its job as one of the eliminative channels (as well as it can).

Avoid constipation. If it *is* a problem, add a bulking agent (like psyllium seeds) to your diet.

Drink at least one-half your weight in ounces of plain water every day. (For example, if you weigh 100 pounds, you should be drinking 50 ounces of water each day.)

Avoid fast foods, which are high in saturated fats, sodium and refined carbohydrates—all bad for the skin.

Get enough exercise. *At least* 10 minutes of brisk walking each day.

Get enough sleep. Most people require 7-8 hours of sleep per night. Arrange your schedule so you get as much as you need, and try not to change your schedule on weekends.

Change your pillowcase every couple of days; use a fragrance- and color-free detergent (the kind used for baby diapers is good).

Skin Care

As painful as it may be for women, *go without makeup*. Even the new "good for your skin" makeup will clog pores. At the very least, remove your makeup before doing anything that's going to make you sweat.

Don't use harsh cleansers on your skin and don't scrub! Wash your skin thoroughly but gently twice a day. Use a mild cleanser and *pat* dry.

Get *some* sunshine but don't overdo. Always use a hypoallergenic sunscreen when going outdoors. If you use one that isn't completely absorbed into the skin, remember to wash it off when you return indoors.

Recipes

Tea tree oil or garlic oil will help clear up a bad pustule quickly—both are antibiotic. Dab a drop on each spot two or three times a day, after cleansing. Tea Tree oil used "neat" or undiluted can be irritating to sensitive skin. If this is the case for you, add 2-5% Tea Tree oil to your normal (oil-free) facial lotion.

Rubbing a fresh strawberry on a spot will also help (if you're not allergic to strawberries); dab fresh lemon juice on pustules twice each day; or rub a piece of freshly-cut pineapple on the spot.

To clear up blackheads, make a paste of lemon juice, milk and oatmeal. Apply to all affected areas (avoid the sensitive under-eye area), leave on for a half hour and rinse off with warm water.

Use Witch Hazel astringent found in the first aid aisle at the store. It's typically 86% Witch Hazel extract and 14% alcohol. The Witch Hazel itself is astringent and with this lesser alcohol content, it's less drying than many other commercial astringents.

An infusion made from Thyme can be used as a toner (see preparations section for "how to"). It is antibiotic. Myrrh tincture diluted in water (1 part tincture to 4 parts water) does the same thing. Chamomile infusion is soothing to irritated skin.

Calendula cream will help heal the skin, especially if you've "picked".

A very useful gel:
  2 teaspoons Evening Primrose oil

2 Tablespoons Aloe Vera gel
1 teaspoon Witch Hazel extract
4 drops Thyme essential oil
4 drops Lavender essential oil

Combine all ingredients well. Massage onto face, neck & upper body (wherever you have breakouts) before bed. Allow it to dry a bit or you'll stick to the pillowcase & sheets.

Internally, there are options but it depends on *why* you have acne in the first place. If the problem is mostly hormonal:
>Women: Chaste Tree Berry (sometimes marketed as "Vitex"), 175-225mg each day in two divided doses.

>Men: Saw Palmetto Extract, 320mg each day in two divided doses.

>Both: Echinacea tincture, 20 drops in ¼ cup water three times per day.

As a blood purifier, Burdock Root decoction, one cup three times daily.

For all-over tonic and system-wide waste removal, either Dandelion Root decoction or Nettle Leaf infusion, one cup three times daily.

If stress is a contributing factor, try Passionflower or Hops infusion, one cup once per day in the evening.

Notes

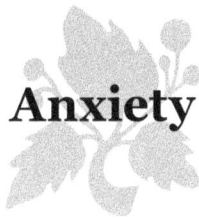

Anxiety

The information here is for general, short-term anxiety. If there is a long-standing problem, please consult a medical professional to determine the root cause and solution.

Make an infusion of any of the following herbs, taking one cup three times each day:
    Chamomile (German)
    Lemon Balm
    Linden
    Oatstraw
    Passionflower
    St. John's Wort
    Scullcap (especially if accompanied by nighttime muscle cramps)
    Valerian (at bedtime only)
    Wood Betony (especially if accompanied by tension headaches)

Seventeenth century Carmelite nuns were famous for their "Carmelite Water", or Eau de Mélisse de Carmes. It was originally developed in the 14th century as an elixir thought to improve memory & vision; and to cure melancholy & depression. Its ingredients tell us that it is calming when taken internally (or as a rub for rheumatism if used externally). One recipe is:
    2 tablespoons Lemon Balm leaves
    1 tablespoon finely chopped Lemon peel

1 teaspoon sweet Marjoram leaves
½ Cinnamon stick
5 whole Cloves
1 teaspoon grated Nutmeg
¾" piece Angelica stem
1¼ cup Vodka

Muddle all herbal ingredients together in a mortar & pestle. Place all in a bottle or jar and add the vodka. Allow to steep 10 days, shaking once per day. Strain the liquid through a sieve, and then through a coffee filter to get all the herbs out. Pour into a sterilized bottle and let stand at least two weeks. One fluid ounce in the morning and another in the evening is a good dosage. It's said the Roman Emperor Charles V (1500-1558 CE) drank this every morning as a tonic.

Fresh Ginger can be added to your meals, or drink a cup of a Gingko infusion with food.

2,000-3,000mg of Ashwaganda taken in divided doses will help balance stress hormone levels.

Ayurvedic medicine gives us the following recipe for anxiety: drink one cup orange juice with one teaspoon honey and a pinch of powdered Nutmeg twice daily.

For an acute anxiety (panic) attack, use Bach Rescue Remedy.

Try to learn relaxation techniques such as meditation or yoga. These can be accompanied by aromatherapy. Put a few drops of the following essential oils in a warm bath, massage oil or room diffuser:
    Clary Sage

Jasmine
Lavender
Melissa (Lemon Balm)
Ylang Ylang

Notes

Arthritis

All arthritis types respond to nutritional support. Your diet should be alkaline, which includes fruits & vegetables with only small amounts of grain and dairy products. It's best to avoid all processed foods. Raw vegetable juices and potassium broth are effective for alkalizing body tissues and dissolving deposits around joints. Try fresh pineapple juice for its bromelain content (do not use frozen juice concentrate – freezing kills the enzymes); potato juice; cabbage and/or carrot juice; and wheatgrass. Be sure your diet is high in essential fatty acids to help prevent arthritis and also for pain reduction. EFAs can be found in fish, olive oil, flax seeds, nuts and avocados.

The sulfur in garlic and onions helps repair cartilage and bones. Eat foods rich in Vitamin K, such as alfalfa sprouts and dark-green, leafy vegetables like kale and spinach.

Osteoarthritis is possibly due to diminished hydrochloric acid in the body, which is necessary for calcium metabolism. Take two teaspoons cider vinegar before meals to restore the acid balance.

Cod liver oil (yes, the same your mother force-fed you as a child) taken two teaspoons in the morning will help increase elasticity and soften fibrous tissue, as well as correcting uric acid metabolism.

On to the herbs:

Arnica gel or cream, topically applied, has been shown to be more effective than over-the-counter pain relievers. Arnica suppresses the various compounds the body produces that causes inflammation.

Boswellia (Frankincense) capsules or tablets will help relieve swelling and inflammation. Follow the instructions on the package. Because Frankincense is a resin, it is difficult to make this herb into something you can take without resorting to commercial preparations. It will extract as a tincture but the resulting liquid may not contain all the beneficial chemicals.

Feverfew and Ginger are anti-inflammatory. Take one cup infusion two to three times a day.

Hawthorn: 100-250mg three times a day will help stabilize collagen.

Yucca extract, 3-6 drops in a little water twice per day, will stop the circulation of toxins to the joints.

Those with Rheumatoid Arthritis should avoid Agrimony and Siberian Ginseng.

For pain relief, apply a Turmeric poultice twice a day, or take Willow Bark decoction or Meadowsweet infusion 3 times per day. You can also make a massage oil of Cayenne, apple cider vinegar & peanut oil. Massage this into the painful areas after a hot bath two or three times per day. Follow with a massage of plain olive oil to ease the sting of the Cayenne.

Essential oils recommended for massage (dilute 10 drops in 1/8 cup of a carrier oil such as almond, jojoba or peanut):

Bay, Cajeput, Cedarwood, Roman Chamomile, Eucalyptus, Ginger, Juniper, Lemon, Marjoram, Nutmeg, Tea Tree and Thyme.

Put a few drops of either Juniper or Melissa (Lemon Balm) essential oil into a warm bath to help cleanse the joints of mineral and acid deposits.

Notes

Asthma

Asthma is a serious condition that, if untreated, can lead to life-threatening episodes. Please consult your medical practitioner prior to embarking on any course of treatment, herbal or otherwise.

First, identify factors in your environment that can precipitate an episode and limit your exposure. Avoid airborne allergens and allergy-proof the house. Eliminate food allergens and food additives from your diet. Follow a vegan diet with the exception of cold-water fish (salmon, mackerel, herring, halibut, etc.). Diet restrictions may take up to a year for you to notice any effects.

Red Reishi (a mushroom) inhibits the chemical reaction that starts an episode, reduces sensitivity to environmental triggers and clears mucus congestion. Start with 30 drops of a quality liquid extract, once daily. Those with more severe cases can slowly increase to 30 drops, twice daily.

Add more garlic and onions to your diet – they are anti-inflammatory.

Make an infusion of any of the following herbs, taking one cup two to three times per day:
    German Chamomile is a gentle antihistamine
    Elder (Berries or Flowers) relieves nasal congestion and
    fever

Ginger opens airways

Green Tea: take at least one hour after any oral medications

Hyssop relieves the feeling of chest congestion

Scullcap prevents allergic reactions

Passionflower calms anxiety & emotional distress, which can trigger an episode.

500mg Astragalus 2 times per day helps strengthen lung function (avoid when fever is present).

120-240mg per day of a quality Gingko Biloba extract is anti-inflammatory and antioxidant.

Lobelia relaxes smooth muscles in the airways and improves the lungs' ability to draw in air. Take 10 drops tincture twice daily in a little juice or water.

Make an infusion of equal parts Coltsfoot, Mullein and Valerian. Take one cup twice per day to ease congestion and expectorate sticky sputum.

Aromatherapy is helpful, especially if used in a steam inhalation. (For a steam inhalation, bring a 2-quart pot of water to a boil and then remove from the heat. Immediately add ten drops of essential oil, bend over the pan while the water is still steaming, cover your head to prevent the steam from escaping and inhale for about ten minutes.) Using essential oils for a chest massage may also be helpful. Use a few drops of the following essential oils, either alone or in combination:

Aniseed

Eucalyptus

Frankincense

Hyssop
Lavender
Pine
Rosemary
Tea Tree

Notes

.

Athlete's Foot

Athlete's Foot is a fungus, generally picked up by bare feet in public showers, such as those found in a locker room. Like any other fungus, it likes moist conditions, so keeping your feet as dry as possible is a good first step. Powder some dried Goldenseal and mix in equal parts with cornstarch. Dust your feet with this mixture prior to dressing and again at bedtime. Goldenseal is antifungal.

Wearing natural fiber socks will help your feet breathe and keep them dry. If your feet sweat a lot, consider changing your socks a couple of times per day. Try not to wear plastic or rubber shoes and never wear the same pair of shoes two days in a row. Switching off allows your shoes to dry thoroughly. If you must be in wet public places (such as at a pool or in the locker room at your gym), wear waterproof flip-flops while walking around and in the shower.

Mix two parts Echinacea, one part Goldenseal and one-half part Poke Root. Powder well and take 1/3 teaspoon in water three times per day before meals.

If your feet have become infected, make a decoction of Black Walnut. Soak your feet in this twice per day. Alternatively, in a small pan of hot (as hot as you can tolerate, but not boiling) water, add 2-3 drops of Myrrh, Tea Tree or Thyme oil, soaking your feet in the liquid two to three times per day. This will not only help kill the fungus, it will calm the itching.

Applying a Comfrey Root poultice for one to two hours each day will kill the fungus. Rubbing a cut garlic clove on the affected area accomplishes the same thing.

Boosting your immune system will help you avoid future episodes. Add plenty of Garlic to your diet; or take 2-4mL of a combination Echinacea/Goldenseal tincture three times per day; or take 2-4mL of an Oregano tincture two times per day.

Notes

Blood Pressure, High

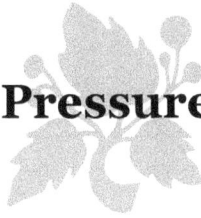

Consult your physician prior to embarking on any herbal treatment. Avoid excess salt or sodium – read labels on processed foods carefully! Reduce excess weight and get regular exercise, such as a 20 minute walk per day. Limit your caffeine and alcohol consumption. Learn relaxation techniques such as meditation or yoga to help combat stress.

Avoid Coltsfoot and Licorice as these can increase blood pressure.

Hibiscus is a traditional remedy for high blood pressure in many parts of the world. One cup of a Hibiscus infusion three times per day may reduce blood pressure by as much as 10%.

If fluid retention is a problem, one cup of Cornsilk infusion two to three times a day will increase urination without depleting potassium levels. 20mL of Dandelion Leaf or Parsley tincture three times per day will also increase urination. (Please be sure to drink plenty of water if taking any diuretic.)

As aids in lowering blood pressure:
Hawthorn: 100-250mg three times per day
Garlic: 600mg of a quality extract twice per day (or add it liberally into your diet)
Passionflower infusion: one cup three times per day if stress is a factor

Other herbs to help the circulatory system overall include: Barberry, Black Cohosh, Buckwheat, Cayenne, Lemon Balm, Onions, Peppermint, Red Clover, Valerian and Yarrow. Try an infusion of any or a combination of these three times per day.

Dark chocolate (greater than 60% cacao) can lower blood pressure by as much as 10%. Enjoy up to three ounces per day.

Ayurvedic texts say that honey scrapes fat & cholesterol from the body's tissues. Lowering cholesterol levels can help high blood pressure. Drink a cup of hot water with one teaspoon honey and one-quarter teaspoon cider vinegar every morning before breakfast.

Notes

Bronchitis

Rest as much as you can – bed rest is preferred. Drink large amounts of liquids such as teas, broths and vegetable juices to thin mucus. Limit sugar consumption (including fruit juice), as this will thicken mucus.

To clear bronchial passages and reduce inflammation, take either American or Siberian Ginseng. Make a decoction and drink one cup three times per day, or take a 500mg capsule three times per day.

1 cup of Elecampane infusion up to four times per day will help stimulate coughing. 1 cup Coltsfoot infusion three times per day will help relieve congestion, but take this for a maximum of one week only. 2mL of a Mullein tincture four times per day will help promote mucus discharge, as will 2mL of a combination Echinacea/Goldenseal tincture four times per day.

To clear bronchial passages and ease breathing, try a steam inhalation (see Asthma for how-to) with any of the following essential oils: Benzoin, Bergamot, Chamomile, Eucalyptus, Lavender, Peppermint, Thyme or White Sandalwood. You can also inhale the steam of a hot infusion of Chamomile (either German or Roman), Elder Flowers or Lemon Balm.

For a dry cough, mix in equal parts: Mullein Leaf or Flower, Coltsfoot, Marshmallow & Anise. Make an infusion of the mixture and drink hot three times per day.

To encourage perspiration (a way to eliminate toxins from the body), try an infusion of: Catnip, Cayenne, Chamomile (German or Roman), Elder Flowers, Garlic, Ginger, Horseradish, Hyssop, Lemon Balm, Sage, Spearmint or Yarrow.

Notes

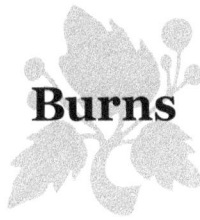

Burns

There are three degrees of burns: first degree is reddening of the skin, second degree shows blisters and third degree may also show only blisters but could also include charring of the skin. Second and third degree burns should receive immediate medical attention, as it's nearly impossible to tell the difference at a glance and both can cause major long-term damage to the affected area, as well as shock, hypothermia and severe dehydration.

First degree burns are what most of us experience, whether it's touching a hot pan or sitting too long in the sun without re-applying sunscreen. The most widely-known first aid is topical application of Aloe Vera gel. This is why so many people keep an Aloe Vera plant in the kitchen – snap off a leaf, squeeze, and presto! Instant gel. Cold-pressed gel is available in bottles at most pharmacies for those without a green kitchen companion. You can also apply Lavender essential oil undiluted directly on the burned area.

Witch Hazel extract will cool a first-degree burn quickly. Dab it on with a cotton pad or keep some in a spray bottle.

If you're *absolutely positive* it's only a second degree burn and the burned area is quite small, a compress made with an infusion of St. John's Wort will accelerate healing and help prevent staph infections. A Blackberry or Raspberry Leaf teabag used as a compress will stop oozing from blisters. In the case of a second-degree burn, always be sure to use a compress of some sort rather than a poultice. You don't want small bits of the herb to work its way into the blistered area.

Calendula gel or ointment, St. Johns Wort oil or fresh Aloe gel will speed the healing process along no matter the degree of burn.

A strong Nettle tea applied topically is a good painkiller.

A fomentation of any of the following herbs will help heal a minor burn: Calendula, Chamomile, Chickweed, Comfrey, Cucumber, Elder Flowers, Plantain or St. Johns Wort.

Notes

Candida/Thrush/ Yeast Infection

A lot of women experience vaginal yeast infections but these sorts of infections aren't limited to women or to that particular bodily area. The usual offending fungus is *Candida albicans* and the infection manifests itself as a white, itchy discharge from the vagina or perhaps a white, itchy coating on the back of the tongue. It can also be a cause of diarrhea.

C. albicans lives in all human beings. For some reason (and they have yet to figure out why) it can proliferate, causing the "infection". As mentioned under "Athlete's Foot", fungi like a warm, moist environment and live on sugar. Diabetic and pregnant women seem more prone to this over-proliferation due to a change in the normal acid/alkaline balance in the vagina. A prolonged course of antibiotics can also cause this over-proliferation.

The cause of over-proliferation must be isolated. It can be as simple as a diet high in processed foods, especially white sugar and white flour; or a lack of exercise and its accompanying deep breathing. A suppressed immune system can cause candidiasis (the technical term for the over-proliferation of *C. albicans*), as can lowered adrenal function.

Avoid yeasted foods (like breads, wine, beer and cider) for at least a week, reintroducing them sparingly. Severely limit any sugar intake - this means fruit, as well. Members of the nightshade family, such as tomatoes, potatoes and eggplant, may also cause problems.

Enjoy vegetables, unsweetened yoghurt, sauerkraut, raw garlic and any rye breads or biscuits.

Douching or gargling will relieve symptoms but not the cause. *C. albicans* will usually respond to an application of cider vinegar. It can be combined with a decoction or infusion of Comfrey, Echinacea, Goldenseal, Myrrh or Sage individually or in combination (2 pints decoction/infusion to 2 tablespoons cider vinegar). Alternatively, add one drop Eucalyptus essential oil to four ounces Witch Hazel extract. Shake well before use and do not swallow if you use this as a mouthwash.

To clear the infection, mix two parts Echinacea, one part Calendula, one part Goldenseal and one part Lady's Mantle. Make an infusion of one teaspoon mixture in one cup hot water and drink three times per day.

Notes

Cholesterol, High

Many factors can contribute to high cholesterol. Sometimes it's a genetic factor: your body may not effectively remove LDL ("bad") cholesterol, or your liver may manufacture too much cholesterol in the first place. Most often, though, it's a result of your diet and lifestyle. Excess weight, inactivity, smoking and a diet high in fat (especially trans fats, which are found in commercially processed foods) can all contribute. Lose 5-10 of those extra pounds by exercising regularly and you may see your cholesterol go down by as much as 10%. Quitting smoking will improve HDL ("good") cholesterol levels.

If cholesterol levels are only slightly elevated, follow your physician's instructions for dietary modifications. This should include ample amounts of garlic and onions, as well as whole grains (oats are quite good), fresh vegetables and fruit, and a handful of nuts each day. Reduce or eliminate animal products in the diet, which are chock-full of saturated fat and cholesterol. Just as the adage says, eat an apple a day. Apple pectin (found immediately under the skin, so don't peel it first) has been shown to help lower total cholesterol levels. Have an artichoke at least once a week. Eat two teaspoons' worth of fresh Ginger with your meals. Liberally add Cayenne, Basil, Oregano and Rosemary as spices in your cooking – these are all rich in antioxidants.

One teaspoon of powdered Asafoetida per day will help lower total cholesterol levels. (Put it in something really sweet like a Stevia infusion to disguise the taste.) 100-250mg of Hawthorn or 300mg of Milk Thistle per day will help the liver convert LDL to HDL.

Fenugreek seeds contain galacto-mannan, which aids in fat digestion. Add two teaspoons crushed seeds to your diet daily (sprinkle them on a salad, for example).

Those with higher cholesterol levels should avoid Gotu Kola.

To help release toxins from the body, put a few drops of Juniper oil into your bathwater or use it in a massage oil.

Notes

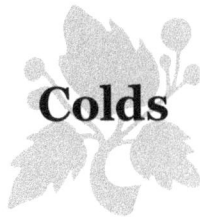

Colds

Just as with Bronchitis, rest as much as possible – preferably in bed. Avoid sugars and dairy products, as these will increase mucus production. Drink plenty of liquids, such as vegetable juices and broths.

Science has confirmed what Grandma has known for centuries: chicken soup *is* good for colds. No, it doesn't get rid of the virus (or prevent you from contracting it in the first place) but may get rid of it faster. It has some anti-inflammatory properties and helps speed up the removal of mucus, easing congestion and possibly limiting the amount of time the virus is in contact with the linings of the nose.

To boost your immune system so you don't get a cold in the first place, make a decoction of Siberian Ginseng and drink one cup three times per day for eight to ten weeks before cold season starts.

If you get a cold, try the following herbal infusions (one cup, three times per day):
    Cinnamon – to break up mucus
    Elder Berries – to break a fever
    Fenugreek – to rid nasal passages of mucus
    Ginger – to ease congestion and stop chills
    Hyssop – as an expectorant and antiviral
    Lemon – to ease a scratchy throat

Slippery Elm – to relieve a scratchy throat
Thyme – to help immune function

Take hot baths or showers to help drain phlegm and detoxify. Add a few drops of Eucalyptus, Lavender, Melissa (Lemon Balm), Peppermint, or Tea Tree essential oil to a bath, or use a steam inhalation with Basil, Benzoin, Eucalyptus, Marjoram, Myrrh or Yarrow essential oils to reduce inflammation and relieve congestion.

Take ½ teaspoon Cinnamon mixed with one teaspoon honey two to three times per day.

For a cold with fever, combine one part each Elder Berries, Peppermint & Yarrow. Drink a cup of hot infusion made with the mixture frequently throughout the day until the symptoms ease.

One of my favorite cold remedies is candied Ginger. It's a pain to make but is very handy to have on hand – most kids will eat it, not knowing you're giving them medicine. You can find fresh Ginger root in the produce section of most grocery stores.

Peel ½ pound fresh Ginger root and slice ¼" thick. Put into a pan, cover with water and bring to a boil. Put the pan lid on, reduce the heat and simmer for 2½ hours. Drain. Simmer in fresh water for another hour or so until the pieces are tender and drain again. Boil 1½ cups sugar, 1 cup water and 2 tablespoons light corn syrup for 2 minutes. Add the Ginger slices. Boil for 1 minute, stirring constantly. Remove from the heat and let cool. Bring to a boil again; reduce the heat and simmer 1-3 hours until the Ginger begins to clear. If it thickens too much, add a little hot water. Remove from the heat and dry the individual slices on a wire rack for a few hours. Roll in granulated sugar and store in an airtight container. Depending on how thick your root was (which will determine how big your final candy pieces are), 1-2 pieces 3 times a day is a pretty good dosage if you're sick, or 1-2 pieces once a day as a preventive measure.

Notes

Constipation

If constipation is a chronic problem, see your physician to isolate the cause. Do not take laxatives on a regular basis. This lessens the ability of the bowels to do their job properly. Barring any serious issues, your diet and/or lifestyle is probably the issue. Ensure you're getting enough exercise to help stimulate bowel activity. Eat a balanced diet of whole foods, including plenty of raw vegetables and fruits. Increase your intake of complex carbohydrates like whole grains, rice, and legumes. Be sure to drink plenty of water throughout the day to help keep stools soft: my water rule is one-half of your body weight in ounces of plain water. So, if you weigh 100 pounds, you should be drinking at least 50 ounces of water each day.

For occasional constipation, add a bulking agent such as psyllium seeds to your diet. Yellow Dock is a very mild laxative: one cup decoction three times per day until you have a bowel movement. Senna (pods or leaves) is a much stronger stimulant. Drink one cup of the infusion twice per day; it's not for children under the age of five or pregnant mothers. 1 cup Hibiscus infusion three times per day will draw water to soften the stool.

An infusion of equal parts Senna leaves, Chamomile flowers and Fennel seeds may help with occasional constipation. Take one cup in the evening prior to going to bed.

Or mix tinctures:

2 parts Dandelion Root
2 parts Cascara Sagrada
2 parts Barberry
1 part Licorice
½ part Ginger

Take two teaspoons of the mixed tincture in hot water in the evening prior to going to bed.

To relieve the muscle spasms associated with constipation, one cup Ginger decoction three times per day; or mix Black Pepper and/or Marjoram essential oils into a carrier oil and massage the abdomen. Abdominal massage helps relax the muscles that support the bladder and intestines to promote bowel activity.

Notes

Cough

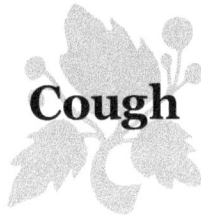

Coughing is due to an irritant in the lungs, whether it's from inhaling dust or another air pollutant; or your lungs trying to get rid of the excess mucus formed by a viral or bacterial infection.

A mechanical way to eliminate excess mucus works well: lie on your stomach on your bed with your torso hanging over the edge (support yourself with your hands on the floor). Place newspapers or a pan below you and then purposely cough ten or fifteen times to expectorate mucus onto the newspaper or into the pan. Do this once or twice a day until you have recovered.

Since you need to get rid of whatever it is, taking a cough suppressant isn't a good idea. If the cough is *really* irritating, taking an expectorant with a nervine may help you relax, especially when you want to sleep at night. *If* your child is over 12 months of age and you want to give them a cough suppressant at night, two teaspoons of honey has been shown to be more effective than the drug dextromethorphan. *Do not give this to a child under 12 months*. Honey contains botulin spores, which adults can handle but infants cannot.

A few infusions for you to try, comprised of equal parts:
Coltsfoot, Horehound and Licorice
Hyssop, Horehound and Valerian
Mullein, Lemon Balm and Valerian

Combine and use one teaspoon mixture to one cup hot water, taken three times per day.

Syrups are a good way to get kids (young and old) to take their medicine. Wild Cherry bark syrup is an old remedy for coughs:
    1 ounce Wild Cherry Bark
    1 ounce Marshmallow Root
    2 pints water

Make a decoction of the herbs, simmering until the liquid is reduced to one pint. Remove from the heat and strain. Return to heat. Slowly add in 1 cup sugar and ½ teaspoon cream of tartar, stirring constantly until the sugar granules are dissolved and the mixture has thickened. Transfer to a sterilized bottle or jar and allow to cool completely before capping. Adults: 1 tablespoon every 2-3 hours; children 1 teaspoon every 2-3 hours. If you are not going to use this on children, you can substitute 1 cup honey for the sugar.

Horehound cough drops can be found commercially but you can also make your own: make a two-cup Horehound infusion (two teaspoons herb to two cups hot water). In a saucepan over low heat, combine the infusion with 3 pounds of raw sugar and four tablespoons honey, stirring until the sugar granules have dissolved. Raise the heat and boil until the mixture hardens when you drop it into cold water. You can add a couple of drops of Peppermint essential oil to improve the taste at this point. Pour onto a greased baking sheet and when it's set but not hard, cut into 1" squares. Once it has completely hardened, the pieces can be dusted with powdered (confectioner's) sugar. Store in an airtight container.

Native Americans roll a Mullein leaf and smoke it like a cigarette to calm coughs. (Hint: this is easier to do when the Mullein is fresh. Take a large leaf, roll it like a cigar and use a piece of twine to hold the roll in place. The interior portions will take longer to dry than the exterior so allow at least a month for the leaf to dry completely. Remove the twine before smoking.)

Notes

Diabetes Mellitus (Type II)

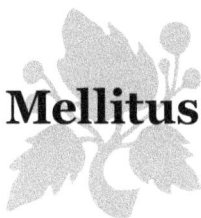

Diabetes can lead to other, more serious issues, so it's best to be under medical care. With your doctor's permission and careful monitoring of blood sugar levels, you can try lifestyle modifications and herbal protocols. If you are insulin-dependent, *do not go off your insulin* unless instructed to do so by your doctor.

Slow metabolizing carbohydrates are extremely beneficial in regulating blood sugar. Avoid processed foods, which usually include concentrated carbohydrates. Whole, unrefined grains such as legumes, bananas, and potatoes with the peel left on metabolize slower and thus don't spike blood sugar levels. Add plenty of nuts, seeds, and vegetables to your diet. Although the body generally responds well to fructose (fruit sugar) as opposed to sucrose ("regular" sugar), you may need to watch your fruit intake if you notice a spike in blood sugar levels.

Be sure to get plenty of exercise to help reduce excess weight and help the body utilize glucose. Try to exercise at an intensity that elevates your heart rate at least 50% for a half hour, three times per week.

Onion and Garlic have shown blood-sugar-lowering activity in several studies, so add these liberally to your diet.

Bitter Melon (*Momordica charantia*) has shown good results in controlling blood sugar levels. The juice can usually be found in

Asian grocery stores. Hold your nose and down a shotglass-full (two ounces) twice per day. Do not use Bitter Melon if you are pregnant or are trying to become pregnant.

Gymnema sylvestre has been used in Ayurvedic medicine as a treatment for diabetes. A touch of the extract to the tongue seems to block the sensation of sweetness, which may cut down on the amount of sugar one consumes. The extract has also been shown to reduce fasting blood sugar levels and to improve blood sugar control. Try 400mg of the extract per day.

Defatted Fenugreek powder has been shown to reduce blood glucose levels as well as to raise HDL levels. Add it to your diet, taking 50 grams of a commercial powder twice daily, or powder 15 grams of raw seeds and soak in water.

Green Tea may help with pancreatic function. Take at least two cups per day.

If diabetic retinopathy is present, take an extract of Bilberry or Grapeseed, 40-80mg three times per day.

If diabetic neuropathy is present, take an extract of Gingko Biloba, 40-80mg three times per day.

Stevia has shown promise in treating obesity and high blood pressure. It also has a negligible effect on blood glucose levels. At 300 times the sweetness of sugar, it is attractive as a natural sweetener. Just a pinch of the dried herb in your cup of tea or coffee will easily replace a teaspoon of sugar.

Notes

Diarrhea

Diarrhea is one way your body gets rid of something it really doesn't like. Often it's a result of food poisoning to one degree or another. Try not to eat solid foods. Replace the water and electrolytes you're losing with sports drinks; or you can drink half tomato juice/half sauerkraut juice. Fruit juices, herbal teas and vegetable broths are all helpful, as well. Be sure to drink plenty of water to replace the fluid you're losing and if the condition persists more than three days, consult your physician to rule out something more serious.

One cup Ginger decoction every two hours will reduce inflammation and lessen the effects of food poisoning (both on the outgoing end and in your stomach).

Three to four cups per day of a Slippery Elm Bark or Marshmallow Root decoction will have a soothing effect on the intestines, as will the same dosage of a Red Raspberry Leaf infusion.

To ease the inflammation and begin the drying process, mix one part Bayberry with two parts Red Raspberry leaves. Make an infusion of one teaspoon mix to one cup hot water. Drink one cup three times per day after meals until the symptoms subside.

3-5mL of an Astragalus tincture two to three times per day will have an astringent (drying) effect. Do not use Astragalus if there is a fever present.

To prevent fluid from entering the intestines, drink one cup of Agrimony or Witch Hazel infusion (made with ½ teaspoon of dried herb) three times per day. Make the same infusion of Bilberry but drink only one cup per day, sipping at it throughout the day. Aloe vera juice drunk one cup per day will achieve the same thing.

Any herb with a high tannin content is going to be helpful as tannins are drying agents. In a pinch, a cup of plain, strong black Tea taken two to three times per day will help.

To relieve the cramping associated with diarrhea, combine equal amounts German Chamomile, Lavender, Peppermint and Melissa (Lemon Balm) essential oils into a carrier oil. Massage this into the abdomen once or twice a day.

Notes

Dysmenorrhea
(painful periods)

It really depends on *when* your period becomes painful. If you have cramping a day or two prior to the start, it could be uterine fibroids which are rarely serious. Be sure to have your doctor check you out thoroughly to rule out more serious problems such as endometriosis or pelvic inflammatory disease.

Cramps are usually caused by the contraction of the uterine muscles to expel the uterine lining. A warm bath or sitting for about twenty minutes with a heating pad on the abdomen can relax these muscles and the cramps will then subside. Stress reduction techniques such as yoga, meditation or massage may also help.

A tincture of Cramp Bark (10-15 drops) in ¼ cup water three times a day for the two weeks before your period starts may stop cramps from starting altogether. Or, 3mL of the same tincture every 30-60 minutes while you're cramping may provide relief within a couple of hours.

Raspberry Leaf is an ages-old remedy for "women's troubles". One cup of an infusion three times per day is the usual dosage.

Two mixtures that may help:
    2 parts Scullcap
    1 part Black Cohosh

1 part Cramp Bark

Or

1 part Motherwort
1 part Chasteberry
1 part Raspberry Leaf

For either, mix together. Make an infusion with one teaspoon mixture to one cup hot water. Drink one cup three times daily or powder all ingredients together and take 1/3 teaspoon in a cup of water three times per day before meals. Adding a pinch of Ginger will help with the pain, as well.

Since the idea is to get the uterine muscles to relax, other herbs are useful to "calm" the muscles. Black Haw, Black Cohosh, Cornsilk and Scullcap can help. Try an infusion or tincture singularly or in combination, taking either a cup of infusion or 5mL of the tincture (in ½ cup water) as needed.

Abdominal massage may also help. To one ounce of a carrier oil, add 3 drops Black Pepper, 3 drops Rosemary and 4 drops Geranium essential oils. Massage this into your abdomen 2-3 times per day until the cramps subside.

Notes

Eczema & Psoriasis

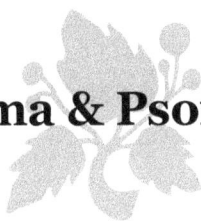

Eczema is characterized by red, itchy skin. It often blisters and then oozes, forming crusts. The cause can vary with the individual, but it is sometimes attributed to allergies, faulty elimination and/or constipation, stress, or a sluggish liver. The patches are often found near joints.

People with eczema should avoid lanolin, coconut oil and products containing coal tar. A gluten-free diet may help.

Eczema may also be due to a metabolic deficiency of lineolic acid (your doctor can test for this). If this is the case, 4-6 capsules of Evening Primrose oil twice per day may help.

Psoriasis appears as red patches that often have a silvery sheen to them and generally don't itch. The patches are often found at pressure points such as elbows, knees, under the bra line or at the waist under the belt. There is no specific known cause but it often runs in families, suggesting a genetic component.

A topical application of Aloe Vera gel is quite soothing. Witch Hazel extract will relieve some of the inflammation; not quite as much as a cortisone cream but it doesn't have all the side effects of cortisone.

Other herbs that can be applied topically to help soothe the inflamed areas are: Chamomile, Chickweed, Oatstraw, Calendula and Rosemary. Especially with Eczema, which can have broken skin, use a fomentation (see preparations) two or three times per day.

Internally, try to regulate your immune system with one cup of Burdock Root, Dandelion Root, or Red Clover decoction or an infusion of Nettle twice per day. Antioxidants will help stop the production of histamines (which cause itching). Berries are full of antioxidants so add blueberries, blackberries, cherries or raspberries liberally to your diet.

To soothe inflammation and relieve itching, an Epsom Salts bath (1/2 cup salts to a full tub) once a day is helpful. Make sure the water is warm, not hot. You may also want to add a few drops of Chamomile, Geranium or Lavender essential oils.

Blue Flag root and Poke Root are an old and effective remedy for psoriasis. Mix one part each tincture and take one teaspoon in water three times per day. Do not overdose as Poke Root is a powerful emetic and has a low therapeutic margin.

Notes

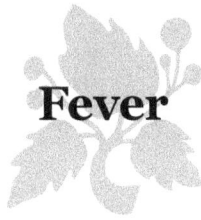

Fever

A fever is usually a good thing – it's one of the ways your body fights infection. Most bacteria and viruses thrive in the normal human environment, but the higher temperatures of the fever kill them. However, a temperature above 103°F (39.4°C) in adults, especially if it doesn't easily come down with treatment, should receive medical attention. Even a slightly elevated temperature in children should receive medical attention as this can signify a serious infection.

If you have a fever, stay quiet and cool. Activity raises your body temperature (as you may have noticed when exercising). Wear lightweight clothing and sleep with only a sheet or lightweight blanket. Many people find that a lukewarm bath for about ten minutes also alleviates symptoms. If you start shivering in the bath, stop bathing immediately. Shaking muscles generate heat. Do not use alcohol to try to bring a temperature down: this is simply too drying for the skin and the alcohol doesn't penetrate deep enough to have any noticeable effect.

My mother used to "sweat" illnesses out of me by making me drink cups of hot tea. As uncomfortable as it is, inducing sweating really works. It stimulates the body's cooling mechanism. One cup of a Hyssop or Yarrow infusion or Ginger decoction four times a day works wonders on a cold or the flu. If you break out in a sweat eating spicy food, consider adding Black Pepper, Cayenne or Horseradish liberally to your diet.

Other herbs you might try to help your body cope with the fever are: Boneset, Burdock, Black Walnut, Peppermint, Spearmint, Catnip (great for children), White Willow, Sage or Thyme.

An ages-old remedy for bringing down a fever doesn't taste very good but works well. Bake a large onion at 400°F for 40 minutes. Remove from the oven and squeeze the juice from the pulp. Mix this juice with equal parts honey and administer 1-2 teaspoons every hour up to eight times per day until the fever breaks.

Notes

Gum Problems

First, do everything your dentist tells you. Brush twice a day, floss and get regular cleanings. Your mouth is one of the gateways to the rest of your body. Bacteria that form there can work their way into your gastrointestinal tract and blood stream, causing all sorts of other problems.

Antibacterial mouthwashes can be made from Clove (2-3 drops of Clove essential oil in ¼ cup warm water), Myrrh (2mL tincture diluted in ¼ cup water), Thyme (make an infusion), or Witch Hazel (two teaspoons extract in ¼ cup warm water). Swish around your mouth for a minimum of thirty seconds after brushing twice per day.

To tighten gum tissue around teeth, make a tea of Comfrey, Sage or Walnut. Swish this in your mouth after brushing. Bilberry tea can be used the same way and is specific for gingivitis.

Green tea is antibacterial and helps stop the conversion of starch into sugar in your mouth. Drink a cup of tea three to five times per day, swishing it around your mouth before swallowing. (This is a good internal antioxidant, too.)

Fruits that strengthen the gum cell walls are: blueberries, blackberries, cherries, elderberries (cook well, first), gooseberries, raspberries and strawberries. Add these liberally to your diet.

Eating an apple gives your gums a nice massage and helps to clean your teeth at the same time. Be sure to leave the peel on. This helps with the massage and most of the healthful chemical compounds are located just below the peel.

Bloodroot has a chemical, sanguinarine, which helps to prevent dental plaque formation. It also blocks enzymes that destroy the collagen in gum tissue. Put 10 drops of a tincture in ¼ cup water and rinse with this combination twice per day.

Alfalfa is very high in vitamins and minerals and is said to help rebuild decayed teeth. Take at least one cup infusion three times daily.

Dentists are divided on whether tooth powder is safe to use. Some say it's perfectly alright, others say it is too coarse and will harm teeth over time. If you want to make your own tooth powder, mix one-half cup of baking soda and one-half cup finely ground sea salt. I add ten drops of Myrrh essential oil (antibacterial) and three drops of Sage essential oil. Sage leaves have been used for eons as a tooth cleaner and whitener. I'm too lazy to powder dried Sage so I use the EO. (If you want to use powdered Sage, use about one tablespoon per cup of baking soda/salt mix.) If you want minty flavor, add up to ten drops of Peppermint or Spearmint essential oil; or spice it up a bit with up to ten drops of Cinnamon EO. (You may have to experiment a bit to get the flavor to your liking as the EOs are strong-tasting.) Mix very, very well to get the oils completely distributed through the powder. Store it in a jar with a tight-fitting lid in the same place you keep your toothpaste.

Notes

Headache, Tension

An occasional tension headache happens to nearly everyone. It can be a result of stress or even poor body posture. Check your posture: when standing, tuck in your buttocks, tighten your abdomen and quit jutting your chin. If sitting, ensure your thighs are parallel to the ground and your head is erect. This will help keep your muscles relaxed. If muscles are tense, many people find relief from hot or cold packs; a warm shower; or even a massage session.

Computers, especially laptop computers, are notorious culprits for headaches caused not only by muscular tension, but eye strain. If you're working at a desktop computer, ensure your monitor is at a height equal to your eyes when you sit up straight. If you use a laptop, look up and out straight ahead of you several times during the hour.

To prevent eye strain, take frequent breaks. Look away from the computer and focus out in the distance for a couple of minutes three or four times an hour. There are even software programs that will remind you to do this!

If stress is a factor, relaxation techniques such as meditation, yoga and biofeedback can be very helpful in both alleviating and preventing tension headaches.

Avoid salt in your diet. Salt can constrict blood vessels, which is one of the causes of tension headaches.

The most widely known remedy for a tension headache is to rub a couple of drops of undiluted Lavender essential oil directly on your temples or forehead – wherever you feel the muscles tight. Diluted Peppermint oil (ten drops in one ounce carrier oil) works well for people who don't like Lavender.

Instead of aspirin, which is synthetic acetylsalicylic acid, take one cup of a Willow Bark decoction or Meadowsweet infusion, both of which contain natural salicylic acid. (If you're allergic to aspirin, don't take this suggestion.)

A tea made of equal parts Scullcap, Wood Betony and Chamomile; or Scullcap, Rosemary and Valerian may alleviate a tension headache. Take one cup as necessary.

If you experience headaches associated with PMS, drink a cup of Ginger decoction three times a day.

For a tension headache associated with stress, Scullcap is a nervine, although some may find its sedative effects a little too strong for daytime use. Chamomile, Lemon Balm, Linden or Oat may be a better choice, here. Try one cup of infusion or ½ teaspoon tincture in ¼ cup warm water two or three times per day.

For a hangover headache, first drink as much water as you can. Undoubtedly, you're dehydrated. Then, take three cups of Dandelion Root decoction, sipping on it throughout the day. This will help clear the toxins out of your system.

Notes

Headache, Migraine

Migraines can often be caused by "triggers". For some, it might be red wine or beer, foods such as cheese or chocolate, the sodium nitrate in hot dogs, or the monosodium glutamate (MSG) in Chinese foods. Overconsumption of salt may also be a factor. If you get a migraine, try to determine if you've consumed a common food or beverage prior to each onset. If so, avoid these triggers.

Feverfew is specific to migraines. Many experts recommend 2-3 fresh Feverfew leaves on a piece of bread; or that you take it in 25mg capsules once per day, slowly increasing to 100mg if necessary, to prevent a migraine from starting. However, if you haven't yet started this regime, try ten drops of a Feverfew tincture in ¼ cup water at the first sign of an impending attack.

Some migraine sufferers swear by Cayenne. Just a pinch of pepper on your tongue at the onset of an attack can stop the migraine in its tracks. The theory is that Cayenne dulls pain receptors.

Gingko Biloba will enhance cerebral circulation and thereby minimize migraine attacks. Buy a standardized extract and follow the instructions on the package.

As with a tension headache, massaging a couple of drops of Lavender essential oil onto your temples may help calm the tension you feel with the onset of an attack. Alternatively, try two drops of Peppermint, one drop of Ginger and one drop of Marjoram essential oil diluted in a light carrier oil such as sweet almond. Massage this into your temples and nape of the neck, then cover your eyes with an ice pack for about ten minutes.

An infusion of equal parts Wood Betony, Valerian and Dandelion root; or one part Alfalfa, one-half part Valerian and one-quarter part Hops taken one cup 2-3 times per day may prevent an onset. For a migraine still in its initial stages, try mixing equal parts German Chamomile, Wood Betony, Scullcap, Thyme and Valerian, taking one cup of the infusion as soon as possible and a second cup in an hour.

Notes

Heartburn/Indigestion

Eat in a relaxed environment and chew your food very thoroughly. Wear looser-fitting clothing. Decrease meal sizes and eat more frequently. Excess weight can be a contributing factor: those extra pounds put pressure on your abdomen, pushing your stomach up and causing acid to back up into the esophagus. Avoid smoking and limit alcohol intake – these can both cause permanent damage to the lower esophageal sphincter. Peppermint and nicotine can cause the esophageal sphincter to relax, causing reflux.

Try an elimination diet: eliminate all suspect foods from your diet for two weeks. Gradually reintroduce these foods until you identify personal triggers. Foods that can trigger a reflux event include citrus fruits, chocolate, carbonated or caffeinated beverages, fatty & fried foods, garlic & onions, mint flavorings, spicy foods, and tomato-based foods.

Antacid herbal infusions of Barberry, Centaury, Chamomile, Dandelion, Marshmallow or Meadowsweet taken one cup when symptoms arise may help.

To protect mucous linings from acid, mix equal parts Irish or Iceland Moss, Slippery Elm and St. Johns Wort. Take one cup infusion three times per day before meals.

Tinctures of Dandelion Root and Gentian Root can improve the tone of the esophagus & sphincter. Take these in small doses: no more than 10 drops in ½ cup water twice per day.

To reduce acidity and encourage healing of damaged tissue, take one cup of a Meadowsweet (not if you're allergic to aspirin), Chickweed or German Chamomile infusion twice per day.

If stress is a factor, see some of the solutions under "Anxiety".

To help with reflux events after bedtime, try raising the head of your bed 6-8" with wooden blocks. Decoctions of Licorice or Marshmallow root, or an infusion of Slippery Elm after each meal and before bed will help, as well.

Notes

Herpes

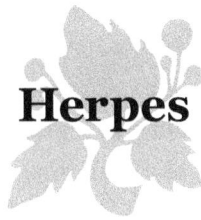

Cold sores are not only unsightly but they itch and sometimes hurt. They are caused by the *Herpes simplex* virus as opposed to the *Herpes zoster* virus which causes chickenpox and shingles. Once any herpes virus gets into your body, it lives there indefinitely, erupting at the most inconvenient times. An outbreak can be triggered by bodily and emotional stress, including the onset of even a minor cold; menstruation; or sunburn - essentially, anything that puts your body out of whack the tiniest bit.

There is no "cure" for herpes but it is possible to lessen the frequency of occurrences. Avoid foods rich in amino acids, which can trigger an outbreak. This includes chocolate! Change your toothbrush after each outbreak of cold sores. The virus can live on the bristles and re-transmit it back to your mouth. Don't share towels or eating utensils for the same reason. If you have an outbreak, don't kiss or shake hands with anyone as you'll transmit the virus to them. Avoid touching the blister or sore and be sure to wash your hands frequently.

If you do have an outbreak, although not an inexpensive solution, mix equal parts pure Lemon Balm *Melissa officinalis* essential oil (usually sold as "True Melissa") and Vitamin E oil. Massage this into the affected area several times a day to clear up the blisters. This solution will also help with genital herpes. Aloe juice and/or Evening Primrose oil may also help.

For Herpes Zoster (chickenpox and shingles), mix equal parts Oatstraw, Nettle and St. Johns Wort. Make an infusion of one part mixture to one cup hot water and take three times per day. This is mild enough to give to children with chickenpox and will ease the symptoms.

Notes

Immune System

Immune means "having a high degree of resistance to disease". Keeping your immune system healthy and intact will prevent a lot of problems. This can only be achieved through a balanced life: nutrition, emotional and spiritual health are all integral parts. A consistent bodily environment is known as "homeostasis" and this is what we seek to maintain. I can't speak to the emotional and spiritual end of things: you'll need to work those out on your own, or with a trusted friend, counselor or advisor.

Immune system maintenance is part-and-parcel of Traditional Chinese Medicine. Western herbalism, because it is so dependent on scientific research, lags far behind TCM. However, we do know that the Western diet with its high fat content, over-processed foods and high sodium content, contributes to many illnesses found in the West but not the East.

Ensuring your diet is full of fresh fruits and vegetables is a good first step. Although I know a lot of people that swear man was made a carnivore, eating a lot of meat just isn't that good for you. If you can't give it up completely, try eating red meat only two days per week, chicken or fish three days per week and go vegetarian the other two.

If you've been on the "bad diet" rollercoaster for quite awhile, your eliminative systems are probably overtaxed and aren't working as well as they could. Detox yourself by drinking nothing but vegetable juices for three days.

Cleavers and Nettle are two of the best overall Immune System tonics. Garlic will help support the cardiovascular system and Dandelion or Milk Thistle will support the liver.

Many have heard, at least in magical circles, of Four Thieves Vinegar. It has its magical uses, yes, but also some medicinal ones. The story goes that during the bubonic plague in France, four men were caught robbing graves and miraculously, hadn't contracted the plague. In exchange for leniency, they agreed to turn over their secret recipe. Many recipes abound but the usual one is:
  ½ ounce Sage
  ½ ounce Lavender
  ½ ounce Rosemary
  ½ ounce Thyme

Steep all four herbs in a quart of vinegar (red wine vinegar being the norm since the story is set in France, but cider or distilled white vinegar will work) for a week, shaking every day. Strain out the herbs. Crush four cloves of garlic and add this to your vinegar. Steep for three more days (shaking every day), then strain.

Other herbs used are Rue, Mint and/or Wormwood. Although there are recipes that use up to twelve different herbs, four is standard: one for each thief. Please don't use Rue if you are pregnant and plan on ingesting your vinegar as it's an abortifacient. Wormwood is mildly hallucinogenic so probably isn't a wise ingredient, either.

This recipe is anthelmintic (expels worms), antibacterial, antimicrobial, astringent, anti-inflammatory and an expectorant. In other words, it helps a lot of problems! You can take a tablespoon of the vinegar every day, or simply use it with a little olive oil as a salad dressing.

Notes

Influenza

Influenza is caused by a virus, not bacteria, so don't ask your doctor for an antibiotic. As preventive measure, try a 500mg capsule of Oregano oil four times per day. Oregano is antiviral.

If you get the Flu, bed rest with plenty of (non-sugary) fluids is recommended. Although I know "misery loves company", keep your illness to yourself. Don't go to work as viruses are spread through the air and bodily contact. Sneeze into a disposable tissue or your sleeve and wash your hands frequently.

A particularly virulent outbreak of influenza during WWI was successfully treated with liquid extracts by the American Eclectic School of Physicians:
    5 drops Lobelia
    5 drops Gelsemium
    10 drops Bryonia

The dosage was one teaspoon 4-5 times per day in water. As all three herbs can be potentially fatal, I wouldn't recommend trying this one at home but its historical reference is interesting. However, all three are available in homeopathic dosages. If this interests you, contact a homeopathic physician for further information.

An infusion of Boneset every two hours will help with the fever and all-over achy feeling one gets during the flu.

To help relieve symptoms, an infusion (one cup three times per day) of any of the following will help:

Anise	to stimulate mucus secretion
Echinacea	relieves symptoms and prevents secondary infection
Elder	relieves symptoms
Garlic	prevents secondary bacterial infection
Ginger	relieves congestion
Licorice	accelerates healing (take for a maximum of two weeks only)
Mullein	soothes sore throats
Thyme	helps relieve cough and fever

Take one cup Cinnamon tea with a pinch of Cayenne every two hours until symptoms abate.

Add Cayenne or Garlic to food, as well.

Garlic, Ginger and Lemon make a great combination for the Flu or a cold. Grate one clove of Garlic, a similar-sized piece of fresh Ginger and juice one lemon. Steep all this in a cup of warm water for 10 minutes and strain. Add a teaspoon of honey. Drink one cup of this every three hours while you're feeling terrible.

Notes

Insomnia

If you are plagued by insomnia, try to figure out the reason why. Ensure your bedroom is cool, dark and quiet. If part of your problem is an inability to turn off your mind, turn some soothing white noise (like the sound of the ocean or rainfall) on low. Practice concentrating on that sound instead of thinking. Avoid caffeinated beverages, alcohol and nicotine after 3pm. While you think you may be sleepy after ingesting an alcoholic beverage, alcohol can actually cause unrestful sleep and frequent awakenings.

A light snack before bed (wheat toast, which contains L-tryptophan is good) is OK but avoid eating a heavy meal at least four hours before bedtime. Other foods that contain L-tryptophan are peanuts, peas, beans, turkey, and pumpkin seeds. Cut back on your fluid intake prior to bed to avoid middle-of-the-night trips to the bathroom.

There are herbal remedies of varying strengths to help you fall asleep. One cup of "tea" (infusion for leafy herbs, decoction for roots) one-half to one hour before bed can help.

Moderate sedatives include: Catnip, Chamomile, Lemon Balm, Red Clover, Primrose, Scullcap & Vervain. Strong sedatives include: Hops, Passionflower and Valerian. (Valerian tastes terrible to most people so take a 50-100mg capsule on an empty stomach rather than drinking a decoction.)

If bad dreams are your problem, try equal parts Alfalfa and Lemon Balm: one teaspoon mixture in one cup hot water about an hour before bed.

Although alcohol consumption can cause restless sleep, an old remedy for insomnia is: steep one ounce Passionflower in one pint white wine for 14 days. Strain. Take one wineglass full (about two ounces) an hour before bed. If you don't fall asleep within a half hour, take one more dose but no more.

Aromatherapy can be a big help with insomnia. Take a warm bath or get your significant other to give you a massage about an hour before bed. Oils that can be added to bath water, massage oil or sprinkled on your pillowcase include: Chamomile, Cypress, Frankincense, Geranium, Jasmine, Lavender, Lemon Balm (Melissa), Neroli, Nutmeg, Orange, Patchouli, Petitgrain, Rose, Sandalwood and Ylang-Ylang. Do a sniff test and find one or a combination that makes you melt into a pile of goo - this is a sure sign of which scent(s) will help you relax.

Notes

Menopause

Technically, menopause is the cessation of monthly menstrual cycles. However, the symptoms start manifesting themselves considerably earlier, during what is known as perimenopause. This can start as early as in the 30's but generally late 40's to early 50's.

First, ensure that all the eliminative organs (bowels, skin, kidneys and lungs) are functioning correctly. Regular short fasts of three to five days on vegetable juices will help, as will eating only fruits and vegetables one day per week.

Supplements of vitamins E and B (particularly B5), as well as vitamin C, will help rebalance the adrenal glands. Parsley, Licorice, Siberian Ginseng and Black Cohosh are specific tonics for the adrenal glands. One gram of powdered Ginseng per day may relieve hot flushes.

At this time, the thyroid gland may not function as well as it once did. Dry skin, puffiness of the hands and face, sensitivity to cold, fatigue and constipation are the usual symptoms. Supplements should include kelp granules or tablets every day, along with herbs high in iodine such as Bladderwrack, Black Walnut, Garlic, Irish Moss, Kelp, Mustard, Nettle, Parsley, Sarsaparilla & Watercress.

Black Cohosh has been shown to be effective for moderate menopausal complaints such as hot flushes and vaginal dryness.

Many women turn to over-the-counter remedies containing Black Cohosh or Soy but don't find relief from hot flushes. Try adding 1.5 ounces of crushed flaxseeds to your diet each day or take one gram of flax oil, which can be found in capsules. Flax has been found to work well when the others won't.

Soy, Red Clover and Hops contain phytoestrogens, which have a balancing effect on the estrogen levels in a woman's body, although these herbs are not a substitute for women who need replacement of the estrogen hormone.

Diuretic herbs such as Cleavers, Hyssop, Parsley, or Roman Chamomile will help to eliminate fluid retention.

Alterative herbs such as Dandelion, Garlic, Burdock or Oregon Grape can be used to aid elimination.

Nervines such as Catnip, Passionflower, Sage and Scullcap will overcome depression and anxiety to some extent, but some women may require a form of psychotherapy or counseling.

Osteoporosis is common in menopausal women, so be sure to get enough calcium in your diet. Calcium-rich herbs include: Alfalfa, Chamomile, Chives, Cleavers, Dandelion, Nettle, Parsley and Raspberry.

Notes

Nausea

Be sure to discover the reason for your nausea. Did you eat something that disagreed with you? Are you on a medication or undergoing chemotherapy? Is this a symptom of a migraine or other illness? Is it always in the morning or at another fairly specific and constant time of day (are you pregnant)? Does it happen with motion (car- or airsickness)?

Several herbs can be helpful, but Ginger is specific to the nausea caused by both chemotherapy and motion sickness - either drink a cup of Ginger decoction in sips before starting out or try a couple of pieces of candied Ginger (see "Colds" for the recipe). Ginger lollipops are available commercially, as well, but be sure one of the ingredients *is* real Ginger or Ginger essential oil, rather than a synthetic flavoring.

Peppermint and Cinnamon are also helpful, Peppermint being more so if the nausea is caused by indigestion or a mild case of food poisoning. Sip a cup of a Peppermint infusion or Cinnamon decoction slowly. There is also a folk remedy that says to determine whether your nausea is "cold" or "hot". If you feel weak or chilled, drink a Spearmint infusion. If you feel hot & "churning", drink a Peppermint infusion.

Many pregnant women turn green at the mention of anything sweet. In this case, try some fresh-squeezed lemon juice diluted in some water. I found a glass of tart (little to no sugar) lemonade taken with a few soda crackers really did the trick. In addition, eating something such as a few crackers or a piece of dry toast before getting out of bed may help. An empty stomach can increase the feeling of nausea.

The lemon juice recommendation is also good for someone with a weak digestive system which can lead to nausea. Take it first thing each morning.

Notes

Sinusitis

Sinusitis can be caused by a number of things: allergies; and viral or bacterial infections of the respiratory tract are the most common.

The first thing you want to do is boost your immune system to fight off whatever is causing the inflammation in the first place, whether it is an allergen, a bacterium or a virus. Garlic helps boost your immune system taken in 250-500mg capsules or tablets twice per day. Add fresh Garlic liberally to your cooking as well - both the pungent smell and the allicin content will help drain your sinuses.

If your sinusitis is caused by a viral infection (such as the flu), take Oregano oil, an antiviral, in 500mg capsules four times per day.

Once you get an infection, an Echinacea/Goldenseal combination (500mg tablets or 5mL combined tincture) four times per day will enhance your immune system and help reduce mucus congestion.

Bromelain (one of the constituents of the pineapple fruit) is anti-inflammatory. Fresh pineapple is very acidic and many people find it irritates their mouth, so take 500mg Bromelain capsules three times a day between meals. Turmeric is also anti-inflammatory: 400-600mg capsules three times per day.

To help clear your sinuses, use Eucalyptus essential oil in a massage, bath or steam inhalation. No carrier oil or water at hand? Simply open a bottle of Eucalyptus oil and inhale deeply.

You can also use Myrrh, Bayberry or Bloodroot as a snuff. Powder each or a combination finely and inhale a pinch up each nostril twice per day.

Another recipe to clear your sinuses: mix one teaspoon fresh ginger juice (juice a piece of fresh root) and one teaspoon honey. Take two or three times per day.

Notes

Ulcer, Peptic

A peptic ulcer is a sore that occurs on the mucous membrane lining the stomach, upper small intestine or the esophagus. Depending on the location, each is given a different name: gastric for an ulcer in your stomach; duodenal for one in the upper section of your small intestine (the duodenum); and an esophageal ulcer for one in your esophagus (and is often associated with gastric reflux disease). Although ulcers were once attributed to stress, spicy foods and an increase in stomach acid production, many ulcers are caused by a bacterium, *Heliobacter pylori*. Stress and the associated increased stomach acid, or spicy foods can aggravate an ulcer.

First, develop an effective stress management program. This could involve yoga, meditation or biofeedback. Get adequate rest; eat small, frequent meals rather than one or two large ones; avoid alcohol, fried foods and smoking.

Despite the old theories, it's now been proven that drinking milk *increases* gastric acids rather than helping calm the pain of an ulcer. Therefore, avoid milk and milk products *except* yoghurt with *L. bacillus*. Avoid the use of aspirins and NSAIDs as these can damage the stomach lining further. Imbibing excess alcohol can also damage the stomach lining.

If your ulcer is caused by *H. pylori*, you will need a two-pronged approach: kill the bacteria and heal the sore. Antibacterial herbs such as Burdock, Chamomile, Garlic, Sage, or Yarrow will help. Drink one cup infusion three times per day. If you find that Garlic irritates your stomach, change to a different herb.

Demulcent herbs such as Licorice, Marshmallow or Slippery Elm soothe an irritated stomach lining or esophageal sphincter. Deglycyrrhizinated licorice is very helpful and can be found in the supplement aisle as "DGL". Chew two to four 380mg tablets 20 minutes before meals. These are considerably more effective than taking capsules.

Drinking one liter of fresh, raw cabbage juice per day in divided doses can effectively heal an ulcer quickly: one study showed total ulcer healing in just ten days.

If the ulcer is bleeding, drink one liter per day of Aloe Vera juice, which acts as an astringent.

Notes

Urinary Tract Infection

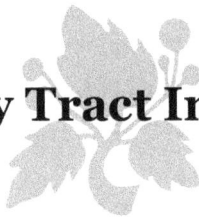

If symptoms do not go away after 24 hours on an herbal protocol, seek medical attention. Urinary Tract Infections are serious: the bacterial infection can travel into your kidneys and from there into your blood stream. If you get frequent UTIs, please consult with your doctor as there may be an underlying issue.

UTIs are caused by an over-proliferation of bacteria in your urinary tract, usually *E. coli*. Everyone has bacteria there; it's just a question of the quantity. Bacteria thrive in an alkaline environment and feed on sugar. Therefore, try to keep your urine acidic. If there's a problem with the alkaline/acidic balance in your urine, drink apple cider vinegar or take hydrochloric acid tablets.

If you do get a UTI, the most common remedy is *unsweetened* cranberry or blueberry juice. Read labels to ensure there is no sugar in your juice, or take capsules. Avoid bladder irritants like coffee, alcohol, chocolate, sodas, citrus juices and hot peppers. Stick to plain water and lots of it.

Uva Ursi is also specific to UTIs as a urinary antiseptic: 500-1,000mg capsules or one cup infusion three times per day. This may turn your urine green but don't worry – there's no harm done.

A Marshmallow Root decoction will increase the acidity of your urine and thus inhibit bacterial growth. Take up to one quart per day.

Diuretic herbs that will help flush out your system include Celery, Cornsilk, Dandelion, Parsley and Watermelon. Again, drink plenty of water to avoid dehydration.

A soothing tea can be made from: Calendula, Marshmallow Root, Licorice Root, Nettles, Peppermint and Uva Ursi. Mix together one part of each, then use one tablespoon of the mixture to make an infusion. Drink two to three cups per day.

Notes

Varicose Veins

Varicose veins are the result of blocked blood flow in veins. Without flow, the blood pools and forms a bulge. They are most commonly found in the legs due to gravitational pressure but they are the same thing as hemorrhoids: they are caused by damage to the valves in the veins and/or increase in blood pressure.

There are only theories as to why they form but one is that obesity is a contributing factor – if you are obese you are less likely to get good exercise, which leads to the loss of tissue tone, muscle mass and weakening vein walls. Therefore, weight loss is highly recommended as is regular exercise.

Avoid standing for long periods. Exercise such as jogging or bicycle riding promotes blood circulation in the legs.

Varicose veins are rarely seen in countries where high-fiber, unrefined diets are normal. Straining during bowel movements puts more pressure on the abdomen, obstructing blood flow up the legs. Therefore, a high fiber diet is recommended. Avoid constipation and use bulking agents (such as psyllium seeds) if necessary.

Add foods rich in flavonoids to your diet. All berries are such, as is Buckwheat, which can be made as a decoction and drunk once or twice per day.

Bromelain (found in pineapples) may prevent the hard and lumpy skin. Since many people find pineapple too acidic to eat in quantity, try it in the extract form, 500-750mg between meals.

Witch Hazel extract (found in the first aid aisle of the store) can be applied to bandages and loosely bound over the varicose veins at night. The astringent action of Witch Hazel may help contract the bulging blood vessels.

An extract of Horse Chestnut is specific for vein problems. Take 15-20 drops of liquid extract in a glass of water 3 times per day.

Notes

Magical

The way you practice your magic is as individual as you are. Therefore, I've only suggested possible herbal combinations and uses. Ritual, and vocal or written spell wording is up to you. That said, I know there are beginners out there, so I'll put in my two cents' worth for practicing magic: accept or discard as you feel it fits with you.

You will probably find it easiest to focus on major issues if, for the most part, you practice your magic in the same place at the same time. When there are other people in the house, a bedroom or bathroom can be easily closed off to minimize distractions. If you're lucky enough to have an extra room to devote only to magical practices, so much the better. You can keep everything in one place and the energies you create will build up over time, making that room one more personal tool (but still cleanse it if someone else spends time in that room … like a repair or pest control technician).

The outdoors (under a particular tree or in a favorite resting spot) is a great place for magic – the Earthly energies will automatically combine with yours. Just be sure that wherever your outdoor spot is that you will not be intruded upon. I have two specific places – one outdoors and one in the house. As much as possible, I'll try to use my outdoor setting but if the weather or amount of passing traffic isn't to my liking, I'll use the indoor area.

Be sure that no matter where or at what time you perform your working that you are focused only on the matter at hand. Some people get ready by taking a bath or shower beforehand to cleanse themselves of the energies accumulated from the day so they go into the working fresh. Others dress in a particular piece of clothing. Whatever it takes to get you "in the mood". It sounds too common-sense to say but I'll say it anyway: since you don't want to be distracted, turn the phone off, make sure you're not hungry or thirsty and use the restroom beforehand. (Nothing interrupts concentration more than a full bladder!)

You may find that animals are drawn to you while you're performing your magic. They can sense the energies moving and either want to feel the energy or add their own – I'm not sure which. Indoors, our cats are always observing me. If I'm outdoors, I notice quite a few birds sitting quietly in the nearby trees and one particular female squirrel has taken a keen interest in me of late. Feral animals probably won't intrude but pets *can* be a distraction. If your pets simply observe, let them be. If they want to "participate", you may find it easiest to close the door on them. Be sure to give them a little extra attention afterward.

I recommend that no matter what someone or something says, that if you don't write your own spell from scratch, you at least personalize what you're doing. Change an herb; change the ratio of herbs if using more than one; change the number of times you do something; change the words; change *something* to make it more "you". Don't be afraid to combine pieces of several spells from other sources into one that you like. What you read in books has worked for others but they got to that particular point by experimentation, just like you're doing. (This is a moot point if you follow a familial or apprenticeship path.)

One thing I want to emphasis: magic is all about *you* and *your intent*. You can have all the tools and herbs you want, but if you aren't focused on the task at hand, it won't work. Magic can be (and often is) performed without anything but your mind. If there is something you *want* to have around, that's another matter altogether.

I almost always light a candle. I *like* candles. Their lighting gets me in the correct frame of mind. Do I *need* one? No. It's tough to light a candle in the car when I want a good parking spot. But if I'm home, I'll generally have one going.

Many people use specific colors for specific intents. Again, this is a personal preference. Some traditions do have lists of color correspondences but if you're following your own path, think about which color you associate with a particular intent. I happen to like blue for harmony, purple for protection, pink for love ... the list goes on. Since I make my own candles, I generally have the 'correct' color around but if I don't, the white taper I bought at Walmart to dress up the dining room table works just fine.

If you do light a candle, be sure to practice good candle safety, too. Never leave a candle burning unsupervised – especially if you have children or pets (I've heard countless stories of smoldering cat tails). If the spell calls for burning a candle for a specified period of time be sure there's someone around the whole while to ensure it doesn't tip over. You also want to keep the wick trimmed to about one-quarter inch so that it doesn't smoke or burn more quickly than the wax.

If you *want* other tools, like a wand, by all means, find one you like and use it. Just know that they are *tools* and aren't indispensable items.

Do you need music? That depends. If you can have music on and not get distracted by it, by all means turn some soothing instrumental music on low. I don't recommend music with lyrics. Whether you believe it or not, they'll creep into your subconscious and become a distraction. If, like me, you start humming along, even to an instrumental, don't distract yourself with it.

Should you write rhymes? Not necessarily. Rhymes are a way to easily remember what to say. (Compare your memory of song lyrics from your youth to a school lesson from the same period. See what I mean?) Many people do use rhymes and even use rhyming dictionaries (yes, such a thing does exist) to get it just right. I come from the school that personalizes *every* spell to the individual situation so remembering *one* rhyme for health (for example) won't work for me. I also can't seem to write rhymes or poetry no matter how hard I try so I gave up trying rather than frustrate myself any longer. I simply state my intention firmly three, seven or nine times.

Many practitioners add a drop or two of their own blood to any mixture they make. It personalizes the mixture in a way nothing else can – you're literally giving a part of your life to it. A finger pinprick is all it takes. Ladies, not to gross you out but your menstrual blood is even more powerful than what you'll get from a pinprick. Again, a drop or two is all it takes. (You can freeze dry your menstrual blood for future use.)

How long does it take for magic to work? My husband came up with a good analogy: you're turning a tanker, not a speedboat. It takes some time. The Universe has to rearrange that energy, which rearranges circumstances to fulfill your desire. Small issues may happen nearly immediately. Others may take a year or more to come to fruition. I did a spell a couple of years ago that I didn't expect to completely manifest for ten years. I structured it that way on purpose to prevent a whole host of unwanted consequences of an earlier solution. Although I'd really like for it to manifest itself much earlier, patience is called for so everything works *right*. I see hints that it's already working, and as intended. Be patient!

I also suggest you work on only one major intention at a time. If you're like me, you have enough going on in your life that you can only truly focus on one intention. More than that, you'll clutter up your mind and won't devote your full energies to what you want to accomplish. If you need to get healthy, work on that first as you won't be able to enjoy anything else until you are. Everyday workings, like for *reinforcing* protection or health, can be tucked into your daily routines without disrupting your focus on a major intention.

Like everything else, practice makes perfect. The more you work with magic, the easier it gets as you go along.

Anger Management

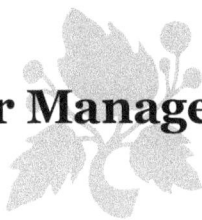

If *you* are the one having anger management issues, meditation may help you get a handle on your anger. Try using Rose, Lavender or Lemon Balm (Melissa) essential oil in an oil warmer as you meditate for their calming effect. Or dress a candle with any of those herbs for use in ritual. (See Preparations for how to dress a candle.)

Make a crown of Violets (use the aerial part of the plant when in full bloom) and wear it while meditating to calm anger. (You can substitute cultivated pansies if you don't have Violets growing nearby.)

If someone you know has anger management issues, the following herbs are useful in spells: Catnip, Chamomile, Lemon Balm, Lavender, Rose, or Vervain. They can be burned as incense, or as stuffing in a poppet (stuff the head – the source of the anger).

Make an infusion of any or all of the above herbs, soak a piece of paper in the "tea" and let it dry. Write the name of the person you want to calm on the paper three times. Burn the paper and blow the smoke in the direction of the person, sending the calming energy their way. Dispose of the ashes in running water such as a river or stream (not the tap), bury them somewhere on that person's property or, with your back to a strong wind, allow the wind to carry the ashes away.

To dispel anger from a given area (for example, after an argument in the home or office), mix powdered Asafoetida and Black Pepper. Either burn this as incense or sprinkle the powder around the area.

To banish anger, dress a black candle with Black Pepper. Perform your spell during the waning quarter of the moon. (Black is almost universally used in banishments. Again, if you don't have a black one, any candle will do.)

Mix together ashes, sugar, and powdered Rose, Jasmine & Sandalwood. I've seen it recommended that you throw the mixture on the person having anger management issues but that would probably make them even more angry. Therefore, place the mixture on a photograph of that person, fold up the picture so the mix sits on the forehead and bury it in a garden, preferably under some flowers generally associated with peace & harmony.

Make a spell jar. The jar material depends on whether you're going to freeze or bury it. Glass doesn't freeze well but plastic will. Fill the jar half way with honey (to sweeten a disposition). Add a good-size pinch of Eucalyptus, Garlic and/or Onion. Write the target's name on a piece of paper, fold the paper & put it in the jar. Turn the jar in your hands (top-to-bottom) at least seven times; ensuring the paper is completely coated with both honey and herbs. Either put this in the freezer (to put the anger 'on ice') or if possible, bury it on that person's property.

Notes

Depression Management

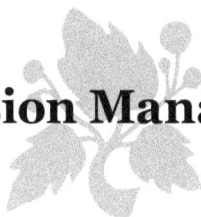

Herbs that raise endorphin levels can be used to combat depression on a magical level. Try either Passionflower or St. Johns Wort in a charm bag. Passionflower is specific to combating addiction so if the depression is related to someone going through drug withdrawal, I'd use Passionflower.

Lemon Balm has a very sunny fragrance and taste and can be used to elevate the mood. For an interesting twist on things, steep one cup (tightly-packed) fresh Lemon Balm leaves in one quart of white wine for two weeks, shaking the container daily. Strain, and use the wine as part of your ritual or spell.

An infusion of Eyebright can be used as a personal eye wash to "brighten one's outlook". For a spell related to someone else's depression, bind a fomentation of Eyebright around the eye area of a poppet for the same results.

Put a piece of Celandine root in a charm bag and carry it with you to lift your spirits. (Many people may experience irritation when handling Celandine, hence the charm bag to keep it away from your skin.)

Medicinally, Oat is used to help depression. It works well in spells, too. You can take a bath: there are a couple of Oat bath products on the market today used for skin issues but they can be used magically, as well. Use Wood Betony in the bath alone or in combination with Oat.

The word "lunacy" comes from the French word for moon, "lune". Use the power and light of the moon to relieve depression. Make a Thyme infusion with rainwater collected during the full moon. Use this infusion to bathe both your head and hair to provide light to your thoughts.

Employment, To Obtain
or Maintain

Carry a piece of Gravel Root (Joe Pye Weed) or a whole, unshelled Pecan in your pocket to interviews or while you're working on your résumé.

Grind a small amount of Gravel Root and Benzoin together. Combine with a little sugar and sprinkle into your shoe before going on a job interview. (Sugar draws ants [who are working], why not a job?)

Use Dill as part of a ritual incense. Other herbs you can use in ritual incense are: Bayberry, Benzoin, Bergamot, Lavender, Pine, Rose, Sandalwood, Sweet Grass and Ylang-Ylang.

Using one or a combination of the essential oils of the above-named herbs, make yourself a personal scent (10 drops total essential oil(s) to one-eighth cup carrier oil), and wear that to your interviews.

You can also anoint a corner of your résumé with this personal oil before sending it out. If, like most people these days, you send your résumé electronically, print a hard copy, anoint the paper and then burn it. Keep the ashes in a crystal bowl near your keyboard, focusing on it when you hit the "send" button.

Two charm bags (either should be green) you can make and carry with you to interviews: combine Sage, Lavender, Dill, Basil & Parsley; or three Cardamom seeds, one Bay leaf and a sprig of Rosemary.

An incense to use as part of your ritual: one part Frankincense, one-half part Basil, Vervain and Mugwort, plus one-quarter part Pansy, Clove and Cinnamon.

If things aren't going well at your job, burn Sweet Grass as incense (if you can) to ensure a happy workplace. If you can't burn incense, bind a piece of Sweet Grass around your office doorknob or twine it around the base of your computer monitor. Or purchase a basket made of Sweet Grass and keep candy pieces in it for your co-workers.

Notes

Fertility

Rice was traditionally thrown at a newly-married couple to ensure fertility. We know now that Rice is bad for the birds and throw bird seed, instead. However, have Rice as one of the side dishes at your reception.

Plan a romantic evening in. Use Olive oil as part of your salad dressing, cook an Italian dish with plenty of Basil, and use Rice as a side dish. Blend one part Rose hydrosol to three parts champagne and drink to celebrate romance.

The Orange tree is a potent fertility symbol: it produces flowers and fruit at the same time. Instead of Rose hydrosol and champagne at dinner, make a Mimosa: one part champagne to one part freshly-squeezed orange juice.

The Pomegranate, because of its many seeds, is associated with fertility. It will take some time as it's not easy, but eat the seeds of an entire Pomegranate during a ritual. You can also drink the juice as part of a ritual.

The Sunflower also has many seeds. Grow the flower in your garden and as the flower opens its face to the Sun, ask it to help. Protect the flower heads from birds with a gauze covering as the seeds mature. Collect the seeds, roast them in a low-heat oven and either eat or use them as part of a ritual designed to bring fertility.

Basil is a good fertility promoter. Keep a plant in a window in your bedroom or drape fresh sprigs on your headboard, replacing them as necessary.

Mandrake is said to come in "female" and "male" roots. Carry a root of the "opposite sex" with you or place under your pillow.

Mistletoe isn't just for the winter holidays. Carry a piece with you or hang it over your bed. (Ensure children and pets can't get at the Mistletoe. The fruit is poisonous.)

Fenugreek is said to be the "plant of increase". While generally used in money spells, make a paste of crushed Fenugreek seeds and massage it into the woman's abdomen.

Ladies, carry a piece of Bistort root on your person (in a bag between your breasts is good). Men, carry a pair of whole, unshelled Walnuts or Chestnuts, or a pair of Juniper berries.

Take a bit of dirt from an ancestor's grave, mix with Roses and burn as incense. Powdered Mullein leaves, appropriately charged, can be used as a substitute for the graveyard dirt if you're miles away from wherever your family is buried.

Notes

Health

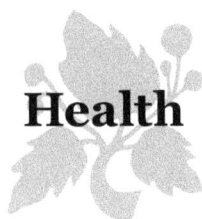

Positive thinking *definitely* affects health. Science has finally figured out that our thoughts and emotions can affect our endocrine, nervous and immune systems, something holistic medical practitioners have known for years. Therefore, always keep a positive frame of mind when working on health-related issues.

Magical herbal healing is very nearly a parallel to medicinal herbal healing. Almost every magical herb has a medicinal quality and vice versa.

The body is one of the most perfect machines there is but it is designed to function at its peak within pretty strict parameters. Illness (or dis-ease) is induced by an imbalance in the body. Stress, cigarettes, alcohol, poor diet, chemically-treated foods and pollution can cause the body to go out of whack quite easily. To heal, you must eliminate the offending substance *and* work to bring your body back into balance with itself. You can't expect to get rid of chronic bronchitis while puffing on your 15th cigarette of the day. Magical herbal healing is another tool you can use to help speed the healing process along.

Consider, too, whether the illness is caused or exacerbated by stress. Examine your daily life to see if things are overwhelming and making you sick. If so, you may want to consider combining elements of both a Peace/Harmony and Health working into one.

"An ounce of prevention is worth a pound of cure." I will repeat what your doctor is continually telling you: eat right, exercise regularly, get plenty of sleep, and practice good hygiene and safe sex.

If something serious does occur, *don't rely on magic alone*. Get immediate medical attention and then *supplement* what the doctor is doing with your positive thoughts and herbal energies.

If there is a specific health issue being addressed, use medicinal herbs for that illness in your spell or ritual.

As an overall boost, or to generally maintain health:

To a full bath, add any or a combination of the following herbs or essential oils: Agrimony, Allspice, Angelica, Calendula, Cinnamon, Eucalyptus, Juniper, Lavender, Myrrh, Peppermint, Rose, Rosemary, Sandalwood, or Thyme.

Oaks are well known for their strength. Use a wand made of oak in healing spells. Carry an odd number of acorns in a charm bag to maintain health. If someone is sick murmur an incantation over an odd number of acorns and bury them under the sickroom window.

Mint is a powerful healer. Place sprigs of fresh Peppermint or Spearmint under the bed, replacing them as they wilt.

Anoint a candle of your chosen "health" color (I prefer red). Rub your candle with vegetable or olive oil, and then roll in powdered herbs, associated with your project, until it's lightly coated. Or, mix essential oils in a carrier oil and rub that mixture on your candle. Burn this particular candle during your spell or ritual. Make up a second candle the same way and burn in the sickroom.

Use Four Thieves Vinegar in a bath or in food magically-prepared. If you choose to use a recipe that includes Rue, don't use this in a food-related spell. Rue shouldn't be ingested.

Place a cut Onion under the bed to help break fevers or under your kitchen sink to absorb "illness". Replace this onion every couple of days. You can also rub the soles of the feet with a cut onion to dispel an illness. Discard the onion after use.

If you're performing a spell involving a poppet, try obtaining a Mandrake root of the same "sex" as the person needing healing. Use that in place of a clay or wax poppet for an added boost to the spell.

Angelica has been used in healing for centuries. Legend has it that one of the archangels appeared in a vision to a monk, suggesting this herb would cure the plague. It did and that's how the herb was named. Add it to any spell as a boost, use it on its own in a bath to wash away illness, or carry a piece of root with you to maintain your health.

Thyme is a powerful antibacterial, as is Rosemary. Burn either one as an incense to purify the air.

Notes

House Blessing/Cleansing

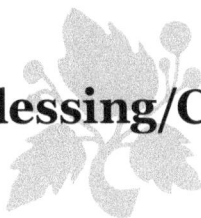

You should always cleanse and bless your new house prior to moving your belongings in. The previous inhabitants may have left some unwanted residual energy. Even if your house is new, all the contractors that have worked on your house have left their imprint as well.

The most widely known house purification is: temporarily disable your smoke detectors. Close all windows and light a bundle of White Sage, ensuring it's smoldering well before starting. Carry the bundle around your home, wafting the smoke into every corner. Allow the smoke to fully dissipate prior to opening the windows and re-enabling your smoke detectors. Some people don't care for the smell of White Sage so Rosemary makes a wonderful substitute.

Some other herbal incense combinations you could use would be:
Juniper & Rosemary
Juniper & Yarrow
Basil, Hyssop & Pine
Frankincense & Vervain
Sandalwood & Cinnamon
Cedar & Pine
Dragons Blood, Frankincense & Sandalwood
Camphor & Cinnamon
Lavender, Mint, Oregano & Rosemary

A periodic cleansing of your house is also in order: I suggest at least once every three months. It will dispel any negative energies left by a disagreement, or the grumpy appliance repairman. A floor wash is a quick way to do this. After actually cleaning your floors, mix any protective/cleansing botanical with a mixture of half salt water, half white vinegar (or put a few drops of essential oil in the water/vinegar mixture). Use a clean cloth or mop to wipe down all your floors. If you only have carpeting, use a sprig of Pine, Cedar or Juniper to asperge (sprinkle) the water around.

Another floor wash alternative is: to one quart warm water add four tablespoons Four Thieves Vinegar, a tablespoon of black salt and three drops of Rosemary essential oil.

To sweep negativity away, use a branch of Broom or Pine. Start in the center of your house, sweeping toward the exterior and then along the wall out the door.

A Fern of any kind, smudged, will form a powerful wall of protection around your home.

If you have a house rather than an apartment, plant a Holly bush near your front door. This will not only discourage negativity in the home, it will please the fairies to no end.

Notes

Legal Matters

Galangal is nicknamed "Courtcase root". Carry it with you into the courtroom. Same for a piece of High John the Conqueror root, Hickory nuts, or a piece of Celandine.

Scatter Calendula blossoms around your house prior to leaving for the attorney's office or courthouse; or carry them with you, either in your pocket or in a charm bag.

Put a piece of Skunk Cabbage in the folder with the paperwork in a case against you.

Take a bath prior to leaving for any legal proceeding, using Calendula, Cascara Sagrada, Chamomile, Turkey Rhubarb or Vervain.

To prevent someone from speaking against you in court: dress a candle in powdered lemon rind or if you have it, alum. Place the candle on top of a photograph of the person (or their name written on a piece of parchment) and envision that person's lips being too puckered to speak.

Cascara Sagrada or Buckthorn (both of the *Rhamnus* Genus) can be used to generate good luck in court. Make a decoction of either and add that to your bathwater. Or, carry a piece of the bark of either with you.

Deer's Tongue is said to give eloquence. If you will be called upon to testify in court, carry a piece with you or ... ask your attorney to carry a piece in his/her pocket as a favor to you.

To win a lawsuit, take two leaves of Sage. Write your name on one and your attorney's on the other (or your name on both if you're representing yourself). Put these leaves in your shoes prior to entering the courthouse. If you worship a deity (or deities), write *their* name(s) on the leaves instead of yours.

Placing a piece of Dill in your shoe before entering the courtroom is said to ensure victory in the case.

Notes

Love, To Attract

Before you can attract another's love, you need to be sure you love yourself! If you're not happy with the way you are, work on whatever you think needs changing first. (If you're not sure, ask a trusted friend what you need to work on.) Once you're comfortable in your own skin, *then* you can work on attracting another person.

Friendships also fall under the "Love" category. There are many definitions of the word "love" and not all of them are of the romantic kind. I love my friends a great deal but certainly wouldn't want to be married to anyone but my husband! Perhaps you need a new friend to hang out with or to do something that you enjoy but your current friends don't. Use a love working to find that new friend.

If you're working on yourself, make an after shower talc. For women: finely powder Lady's Mantle, Jasmine, Lavender, & Lemon Balm. Combine equal parts with cornstarch, rice powder or arrowroot powder. Throw in a pinch of Orris Root and another pinch of Chocolate powder. Test on your skin (crook of your elbow is a good spot) to ensure nothing irritates you then put in a tightly sealed container. Use this after each bath or shower. For men: replace the Named botanicals with Cinnamon, Lemon Peel, Peppermint, & Rosemary. In a pinch, you can combine just Orris Root powder with cornstarch.

To attract a new friend, serve lemonade at a party.

To keep someone faithful to you, steep a half ounce of crushed Cumin seeds or crushed Dill seeds in a bottle of red wine for 2 weeks. Strain out the seeds before serving to your loved one.

Showy flowers not only attract bees, they attract love as well. Use Gardenia, Hibiscus, Hyacinth, Orchid, Rose or Violet flowers. Place them on your altar or carry them with you. Polynesian women wear a Gardenia behind their right ear to indicate they're available.

Sprinkle Basil around your home to mend lovers' quarrels.

Take a bath and use either the herb or essential oil of Birch, Cardamom, Ginger, Lavender, Palmarosa, Rose, Rosemary, Vanilla, Vervain, Yarrow or Ylang Ylang.

Anoint a candle with one of the above herbs or essential oils and use it in your ritual or spell.

Everyone blows on a gone-to-seed Dandelion as a child. Some make a wish and allow the seeds to scatter their wish to the wind. Others say that the number of times they have to blow to completely clear the head is the number of years until they meet their true love. Revive this tradition: blow on a Dandelion to carry your love messages.

Carry a piece of Copal or a Vanilla bean in your pocket or in a charm bag.

Pierce Juniper berries and string them into a necklace. Wear this to attract love.

Just as Catnip draws cats, it can draw lovers as well. Make an infusion of Catnip, Lavender and Vervain. Use the infusion in your bath prior to going out with friends.

If there's someone you'd like to get to know "a little better", carry a piece of Wood Betony with you on the evening you make your proposition.

Make a salad and include Chickweed, Endives, Lovage and Oregano as part of the ingredients. Serve Red Beets as a side dish. Season your main dish with Marjoram, Oregano, Rosemary, or Thyme. Serve Apple pie for dessert.

Nothing says "love" to most as chocolate. Serve your lover a cup of piping hot chocolate, add a dollop of whipped cream and sprinkle liberally with Cinnamon.

Back in 1965, the Searchers had a hit with "Love Potion #9". Traditionally, you would make a strong infusion with nine herbs of love and serve it as an aphrodisiac. If you want to be true to the song, it will have to smell "like turpentine" and "look like India ink". Dragon's Blood or Benzoin would make it smell terrible and Juniper berries would give it a dark color.

Notes

Mental Powers, To Strengthen

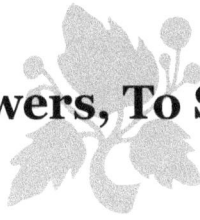

Do you have trouble concentrating? Or perhaps you're not absorbing that school subject as well as you'd like. In addition to learning to meditate which will help your concentration, there are magical things you can do to strengthen your mental abilities. *Anyone can learn anything.* It's a question of perseverance. I have a friend who is dyslexic, making it difficult for him to read. However, he still reads 500-page novels; he taught himself to concentrate hard on each word until it made sense to him.

This holds true for psychic powers as well. Developing a psychic ability is no different than learning an unfamiliar and/or difficult subject. I believe everyone is born with some psychic ability. The trick is learning to concentrate and recognize it.

If you're having trouble concentrating or learning something difficult the first thing you need to do is get rid of outside distractions. Remember, magic is only a tool and you have to help yourself. Pick a spot where concentration is what you do in that place. Don't make it too comfortable – the easy chair in the living room isn't the best idea. I wouldn't recommend the kitchen table, either, unless that's the only place you have. Traffic to and from the refrigerator can be distracting, not to mention that last piece of cake calling your name. Ensure the TV, radio and phone are off if they are a distraction. Tell the family that when you're in that spot that you are not to be disturbed unless it's a life-and-death matter.

Once you've created a "concentration" space, you can start your herb magic.

My personally-tested candle is one anointed with Rosemary essential oil. It got me through the science part of my Master Herbalist course. Or, mix powdered Rosemary with Benzoin and burn it as incense when you're meditating or need to concentrate.

Drink a cup of Sage or Spearmint infusion. For some "oomph" add a couple of drops of Vanilla extract or a pinch of Nutmeg. Grape will help with concentration but fermentation probably won't, so eat grapes or raisins; or drink grape juice instead of wine.

Coffee is well-known as a stimulant but can also be used to strengthen psychic powers. Try Hazelnut Coffee for an added boost. Or, as many witches already know, a Mugwort infusion is a boost, as well. The scent of Wormwood is said to increase psychic powers but it can also just get you high. Use with caution. Ground coffee can be used alone or combined with other herbs to make incense.

Dandelion Tea can be used to strengthen psychic abilities. Its bodily-tonic qualities help here – it cleans out "blockages".

Chew Celery seeds as an aid to concentration or munch on Celery stalks while you're studying … this is a healthy snack, too.

Clary Sage (clary = clear) can be used to help with learning – no matter what you're trying to learn. Try massaging a few drops of the essential oil diluted in a carrier oil onto your forehead, in the spot between and just slightly above your eyebrows. This is the

Brow (or Third Eye) Chakra and is associated with meditation, intuition and learning.

Bay, Lemongrass and Yarrow herbs can be combined as incense or use the essential oil combination (diluted, of course) to anoint your Brow Chakra. Or, rub Honeysuckle flowers on your forehead.

Make an infusion of Eyebright and use it as an eyewash to "open your eyes" to what you want to learn.

An infusion of Flaxseeds, Chamomile flowers or Peppermint leaves, or a decoction of Cinnamon is good to drink before starting whatever it is you need to concentrate on.

Add Celery, Dill, Lemongrass, Mustard, Rosemary, Sage, Savory or Thyme to your spell-infused cooking.

Notes

Peace/Harmony/Happiness

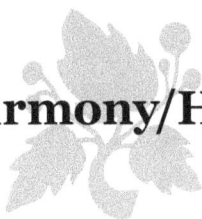

Have you ever been around a person who is so negative they bring you down with them? Do all the little "oops" during the day build up until you're as grumpy as a bear by 5pm? Conversely, have you ever heard someone laugh and find yourself smiling even if you don't know what was funny? Is there a person you like to be around because they're such a positive/happy person? Look at the difference in the energies being produced.

Workings for Harmony and Happiness also can be applied to common, everyday stress. Today's hectic world puts stress on us both physically and emotionally, and takes its toll. If you find yourself rushing around to take care of work, your family and your home seemingly with no time to breathe, first make an appointment with yourself for yourself! You can't be effective in everyday life if you're burned out. Take an hour twice a week to do something just for you … not for anyone else. During a part of just one of those hours, try a working designed to bring Harmony into your life.

You can help yourself maintain a good thought by writing down all the things that make you happy and keep the list on you, or pinning up photos where you'll see them often. My personal happy thoughts are my wonderful husband, our crazy cats and our beautiful mountain home.

Do things that make you happy, too. Listen to music that makes you want to dance – even if you have two left feet and can only tap your foot out of time to the music. Watch a funny movie. Read a least one joke a day guaranteed to give you a belly laugh. (Laughter truly is the best medicine. Science has found that a good belly laugh helps keep your lymphatic system flowing smoothly.) If the news depresses you, don't watch it! In other words, be proactive about creating that harmony or happiness.

Pick your herb(s) and method, and start changing your corner of the world. I think after awhile you'll notice that negative person isn't around anymore or all those little "oops" become small potholes instead of gigantic sinkholes in the road of life. Somehow all the demands your time won't seem so overwhelming, either.

Bowls of nice-smelling potpourri placed strategically throughout your house or on a corner of your desk will help calm the atmosphere and the people smelling the herbs' aroma – especially when magically charged. Try a combination of Gardenia, Jasmine and Lavender; or Frankincense, Myrrh and Sandalwood.

Plant Hyacinth bulbs near the entryway to your house to encourage a happy home.

Real estate agents understand that some aromas imply comfort & happiness. They often suggest that a homeowner bake something just before a house is being shown to induce comfortable feelings in prospective buyers. You don't need to be a master pastry chef: put a handful of Cinnamon sticks and about half that amount of Cloves into a pot of water. Allow this mixture to simmer on the stove for a couple of hours until the aroma permeates the house. It will trigger peaceful feelings in the inhabitants.

Vervain is a medicinal tonic and in this case, can be a tonic for your soul. It is a light, airy-looking plant with small, blue blossoms that always looks happy. Grow it around your house so its happiness protects the house. Make an infusion of Vervain and use it to wash negativity away, whether in your home or in yourself.

Dove's Blood ink isn't made with the blood of a real bird. To a small bottle of red ink, add ten drops of Rose essential oil. Write the full names of your family on a piece of pink paper with this ink and bury the paper under your front steps or immediately to the side of your front door to ensure everyone in the family stays happy.

Burn an incense of Yarrow and Passionflower to dispel negativity.

Look under the medicinal section on Anxiety for herbs designed to calm folks and incorporate those into your spell. Wood Betony also makes a good addition to any incense combination. So does Coltsfoot (which "calms" coughs).

Notes

Prosperity

Prosperity can mean different things to different people. The most usual definitions are: luck, money and success. I'll address all three.

Luck is "to prosper or succeed especially through chance or good fortune". In other words, being at the right place at the right time through no fault of your own. If you're having a run of bad luck, use magic to change it to good.

Money isn't necessarily having the actual currency in your wallet or the electronic equivalent in your bank account. "Money" is having the financial ability to get what money can buy. Let me say that magic won't make twenty dollar bills mysteriously appear in your wallet. Be on the lookout for a different manifestation: a new job or raise in pay, a less-than-expected bill or an unexpected gift.

Success can be "the favorable termination of a venture" or "the attainment of wealth, favor or eminence". So, completing a home improvement project could be a success, or you could succeed at your chosen profession.

To achieve success in any undertaking, take a bath using one or more of the following herbs or essential oils: Basil, Benzoin, Cedar, Cinnamon, Clove, Fenugreek, Frankincense, Ginger, Lemon

Balm, Patchouli, Red Clover, Sandalwood, Spearmint, Vervain or Vetivert.

Anoint a green candle with one of the above herbs or essential oils and burn it during your ritual or spell to draw money. Green is almost universal in its use in money spells.

To attract prosperity, wrap a piece of paper on which you've written your wish around a magnet. Magnetite, a naturally-magnetic stone, is even better than a refrigerator magnet. (Don't use hematite as this will lose its magnetic property over time.) Dress the paper with your choice of prosperity oil. Secrete your paper/magnet in with your business papers, in a cash register for business success, in your toolbox to complete a home improvement project, or in with your study items for school achievements. If you're trying to attract financial gain, use a dollar bill instead of plain paper.

Basil is specific for "drawing" as in "come hither". Carry a basil leaf in your wallet or anoint your business card and/or résumé with a drop of the essential oil. If you have a brick-and-mortar business, put a leaf in your cash register; powder the dried leaf and sprinkle it at your door; or anoint your door frame with the essential oil.

Bobbing for apples on Hallowe'en isn't just a fun game. Supposedly, the first to come up with an apple in his or her mouth will have good luck for the coming year. (Remember, Hallowe'en is also Samhain, the beginning of the Celtic New Year.) Therefore, eat an apple as part of a "good luck" ritual.

When one is successful, it used to be said that one was "rolling in clover". Make an infusion of Clover (usually Red but any color will do) and add it to your bathwater. Be sure to completely immerse yourself at least once so you're "rolling in clover", too.

Encase a 4-leaf clover in beeswax and carry it in a moleskin pouch for luck in games.

Corn is a lucky plant. Take several pieces of cornsilk from the largest ear of corn you can find (so you have long strands of silk). Tie nine knots into the silk as you envision your goal. Carry that knotted cornsilk in your pocket until your goal is achieved, and then burn it. Bury the ashes under an Oak tree or Holly bush.

To bring good luck to you: put salt and pepper on onion skins (the thin outer layer) and then burn them on a Friday morning.

Carry a piece of Vetivert root or a single acorn for success in all undertakings.

As mentioned before, Fenugreek is the "plant of increase". Use the seeds as part of your spell or crush the seeds and make a decoction to drink or use to anoint things.

Bergamot, the distinctive scent in Earl Grey Tea, is a traditional ingredient in fortune and money spells. Use the essential oil in a personal after-bath talc made with cornstarch and/or arrowroot powder. However, be careful. Bergamot is photo-sensitizing so stay out of the sun when using this. Alternatively, drink a lot of Earl Grey Tea.

If you need some luck in your home, plant Hollyhocks by the door. They are favored by the fairies that bring luck with them. Use Jasmine or Peppermint as a floor wash to invite luck into your home.

To attract prosperity, take a bath and use specially-prepared bath salts. For Luck, dye your salts yellow or orange and add a few drops of Jasmine and Vervain essential oils. For Money, dye your salts green; add several drops of Bayberry and one drop of Sandalwood essential oils.

If you make up any liquids (oil combination, washes, etc.) to draw Money, add a piece of magnetite and a few iron filings to the bottle.

Although the odor may repel people, carry a piece of Horseradish in your purse to that New Year's Eve party. If you do so, you will not run out of money in the coming year.

Carry a handful of hazelnuts in your pocket to ensure luck: a naturally-joined pair is even more powerful.

Notes

Protection

Protection can be for many things: guarding against psychic or physical attack, injury, accidents, watching over valuables, etc. Magical protection will also help increase your body's natural defenses (your immune system).

I find it very interesting that the incenses burned in religious rituals are nearly all made up of herbs used not only for protection but for health! Incense, or fragrant smoke, has been a part of religious rituals for as long as there has been religion. The Maya used incense in their rituals over 5,000 years ago; residue of the burning of Copal has been found on ancient altars. Frankincense & Myrrh were given to the baby Jesus by the Magi[1]. Back in the 1300's when the Black Plague was devastating Europe, the (Roman Catholic) Church used the smoke of resins with healing properties in their Masses. (They didn't know it then but most resins are antibacterial.) Since the incense was sweet-smelling, church attendees took long smells, drawing the smoke deep into their lungs which moved from there into the rest of their body. I haven't seen any research that indicates the church-going population was less-affected but it certainly didn't hurt. Those same incenses are still in use today.

---

1   "Magi" is from the same root in the Greek language as "magic". The use of the word Magi to describe the men who visited the baby Jesus was in Latin versions of the Bible until the King James Version (first published in 1611), where it was variously translated to "wise men" and "sorcerers".

Personal protective magic creates an aura around you that, to the unseen world, projects an air of confidence and a "don't mess with me" attitude. That aura forms a shield. Practicing protective magic doesn't mean nothing will ever happen to you. However, it will *help* keep out negative or foreign energies.

Protective magic is very similar to cleansing or purification magic. You can use most of the protection herbs to cleanse your house, office or yourself. Cleansing is driving away negative or foreign energies which is also the focus of protective magic. You should perform a purification working on any new home prior to bringing your belongings inside. I heartily recommend that you cleanse any magical tools and your personal magical area on a regular basis. Family, guests, even the appliance repairman leave their own energies around that may or may not be beneficial to your workings.

Hyssop, Lavender, Patchouli and Rue are considered "botanical guardians". Planting Hyssop or Lavender around the perimeter of your house will keep nasties out. A bit of dried Patchouli or Rue slipped into your strongbox will keep your important papers safe.

Cedar trees will protect your house from lightening, or hang a bough over the doorway to protect the interior of the home. Use the smoke of Cedar incense in purification workings.

To protect yourself or a loved one while sleeping, tie a sprig of Mugwort or St. John's Wort over the bed with a red cord.

Garlic is well-known as protection against vampires but it's a good overall protective herb, as well. Add it liberally to your diet and you'll not only reap the immune-boosting benefits, you'll infuse your body with its protective qualities. Since you're going to cook with it anyways, keep a few cloves hung somewhere in your kitchen to protect not only your food but the chef.

White Sage is well-known as a cleansing & purifying herb but an incense of Dragon's Blood, Sandalwood and (sea) salt burned and the smoke wafted throughout your house will also cleanse away any negative energies. It will also form a protective shield. A bundle of dried Rosemary is a good substitute for White Sage.

A decoction of Vetivert root or infusion of Rosemary or Vervain can be used to bathe not only yourself but ritual items.

Use the smoke of an incense including Basil, Juniper, Wood Betony, Wormwood or Yarrow to form a protective shield. If you don't mind the smell, add a pinch of Asafoetida in there, as well.

The Potawatomi burn Cedar on coals for purification. The Shusurap use Wormwood to fumigate their house and to keep germs away.

Salt is a powerful magical and spiritual protector. It is preferable if you use either sea salt, rock salt or at least kosher salt (which has been blessed). Use salt as close to its natural form as possible without having been processed, although regular iodized table salt will do just fine in a pinch. Add it to baths for cleansing and to produce a psychic shield. You can also sprinkle it around the outside of your house to form a psychic barrier. If you choose to sprinkle salt around outside, *don't get any on the plants* unless your yard is the ocean. Salt will kill land-based plants.

Notes

Sleep

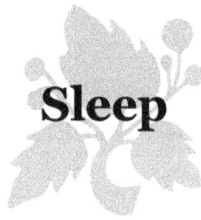

As with everything else, ensure you've done the mundane things to solve your problem before and in addition to using magic. Check the medicinal section "Insomnia" for tips to help you sleep.

The Chamomile, Passionflower or Scullcap tea you drink before bed can be infused with magical intentions.

If you follow a religion, place a sprig of Chamomile inside the main book, e.g., Bible if you're Christian or Book of Shadows if you're Wiccan; and sleep with that book under your pillow.

Make a dream pillow of Chamomile, Hops, Lavender, Peppermint, Rosemary and/or Thyme. Use the herb(s) whose aroma makes you feel calm. Then place it near your pillow at night.

An alternative dream pillow is St. John's Wort & Thyme to prevent nightmares.

While the Poppy is heavily associated with the drug Opium (which does make one sleepy), there's no need to use an illegal drug. Simply grow some decorative poppies in your garden or in a planter on your deck and place their fresh blossoms on the pillow next to you.

Anoint your pulse points (temple, side of neck just below the ear, wrists, behind the knees, and ankles) with an essential oil combination diluted in a light carrier oil such as cocoanut or grapeseed. Try Bergamot, Chamomile, Cypress, Jasmine, Lavender, Rose and/or Ylang Ylang.

If nightmares are troubling you (and you're sure they're not coming from the outside), burn Benzoin as an incense prior to bedtime. Benzoin is an astringent resin and will "dry up" negative energies. Alternatively, place a sprig of Wood Betony or Thyme under your pillow.

Place a number of Bay leaves equal to the number of hours you want to sleep under your pillow. This is particularly effective if bedwetting is an issue.

A sprig of fresh Rosemary placed under the bed will improve sleep & prevent nightmares.

Combine Chamomile oil, fresh Valerian root, dried Poppy pods & flowers, fresh St. John's Wort, fresh Rose and dried Dill. Use this combination in a poppet or make an infused oil for frequent/ future use.

Notes

Theft

In addition to the magical "Protections", you can do many things to prevent theft:

Bury a piece of Licorice or Vetivert root at the corners of your property; plant Hyssop or Juniper near your house; sprinkle Four Thieves Vinegar around the perimeter of your house; or hang Garlic, Juniper, Rosemary or Elder over your front door. If your climate will support them, Aspen trees make great protectors.

Place pieces of Blessed Thistle in the corners of your house and at the doorways to ward off thieves.

If something has been stolen, wear a piece of Vervain, or use it in incense during your ritual to recover that item.

To protect a specific item, string Juniper berries on a red cord. Wind the cord around the item you want to keep safe: e.g., your jewelry box or the rearview mirror of your car.

To protect specific objects, sprinkle them with an infusion of Marjoram. To discourage thievery in general, sprinkle that same infusion around the interior perimeter of your home (or office).

Make a charm bag and fill it with Caraway, Frankincense, Juniper, and one Aspen leaf. Hang it over the door to your house.

If it's too late and something has been stolen from you, the Pow-Wow method of finding a thief is to collect a Sunflower during Leo. Put it under your head at night and you will see the thief in your dreams.

To find a thief: bend a Juniper branch until it touches the ground and weigh it down with a heavy stone, all the while calling out to the thief. He or she will be forced to return the stolen goods. Once the goods have been returned, release the branch and return the stone to where you found it.

To return what was stolen, combined dried Mullein, powdered Garlic, dried Calendula, dried Bindweed and salt. Throw this in the fire while calling for the goods to be returned.

The Paiute use an infusion of Datura to find lost objects.

Notes

Travel

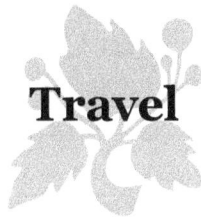

To prevent fatigue while travelling, carry a piece of Mugwort. To prevent "headaches", carry Feverfew blossoms in a charm bag.

To ease your way, carry a piece of Mint on your person.

Place a piece of Comfrey root, Sea Holly root or a few Lavender blossoms in your luggage to prevent its loss.

To protect your car, tape a Plantain flower (it looks like a spear coming up from the flat-to-the-ground leaves) to the visor or just behind the rear-view mirror. A cat's whisker will offer the same protection.

To ensure a safe trip, make up a charm bag of Caraway, Comfrey, Juniper, Mugwort and Rosemary. Carry it on your person or hang it from your car's rearview mirror.

If you're travelling by car, put three Holly leaves, one clove Garlic, one sprig Cedar and one chunk of Dragon's Blood in a small box. Put this in the glove compartment of your car.

To protect a loved one who is travelling, you will need: three candles of your choice of protection color (I prefer purple for this purpose but any color that says "protection" to you will work), a photo or personal article of that person, Sandalwood essential oil, and your choice of meditation incense. Lay the photo (or personal article) flat on your altar or work table. Anoint the candles with the essential oil and place them to the left, top and right of the photo. Place your incense burner below the photo. Light the incense, and then light each candle in the order left, top and right. Visualize a protective aura around that person. Insert your verbiage here as desired. You can let the candles burn out or if the person is travelling for more than one day, burn a little each day they're on the road, snuffing them out in reverse order as lighting (right, top, left). Never blow out a candle. You will blow away all the good intentions.

Sew a 4-leaf clover into your clothing to guard against danger when travelling.

From Bavaria: Pick Daisies between noon and one o'clock on St. John's Feast Day (June 24), wrap them in paper & carry with you for protection on business trips.

If you're hiking, use a walking stick made of Juniper to bring good luck. (This is particularly effective if you're walking in the woods looking for something specific.) A sprig of Juniper in your hat will prevent blisters from forming.

To protect yourself while traveling, powder Vervain & Vitex together. Carry this powder in a hollow ring or locket which has been inscribed with the symbols for Virgo, Mercury & Saturn.

Notes

Grow Your Own

I am a firm believer in growing your own herbs. It provides you with a connection to the plant that just can't be achieved when using dried herbs purchased from someone else. Even if you live in the heart of a big city, in an apartment or condominium without a balcony or patio, you *can* grow herbs yourself.

Most herbs aren't picky growers at all. With only a moderate amount of attention, you can have a jungle of very useful (and some very pretty) plants. Since you're only growing for yourself (and perhaps your family) one, two or three plants should provide all you need.

If you're lucky enough to have space for a garden plot (even a small one), read up on what will grow in your climate. (Unless you live in the desert with room for a large tree, plan on purchasing your resins, though!) Also read up on companion planting: this is growing plants near each other (or even in the same pot), that are beneficial to each other. One example is growing Garlic underneath your Rose bushes. Garlic keeps aphids away.

Be cautious when planting any herb in the Mint (Lamiaceae) family. These spread rapidly via rhizomes (underground) and will take over the space you allot to them, and their neighbor's, too. If you're short on space, consider planting these in pots or build them their own beds, blocking them from their neighbors.

Since most people don't have the luxury of space for an outdoor garden, I'll talk about what you can grow in pots. Some are easier than others.

For each herb, you want a pot about 10 inches in diameter. Ensure it has a drain hole in the bottom and if it doesn't come with its own drain saucer, pick up a cheap plate (of the appropriate size) at a flea market for use as one. Use commercial soil that has been formulated for use in pots. This will provide enough sand to keep the soil aerated and won't allow it to pack down. Even with the drainage hole, I *always* put some gravel in the bottom just in case my hand slips and I overwater.

If you plant seeds, you'll need to thin them when the plants have two sets of leaves on them to prevent overcrowding in the pot. Read the back of the seed packet & look at photos of mature herbs to determine how many plants per pot you can support.

If you're in a hurry, or your plant may not germinate well from seeds, check your local garden center from February to April (depending on your climate). This is when they'll have the best stock of herb plants.

Now, which herbs to grow? Which are your favorites? If you cook, which ones do you use the most in the culinary sense? Which ones do you find the most useful for *you*, in both a medicinal and magical sense? Start with ten. You can always add more when you're comfortable being a gardener.

The following herbs like as much sun as they can get. If you don't get a lot of sun at your place, you might consider investing in a grow light.

Basil: grows easily from seed. However, it needs pinching on a regular basis or will get very leggy. Seems to be happiest in a sunny kitchen window – right where the cook can get to it!

Bay: is a small tree when it gets going so be sure you have an even larger pot to put it in when it matures. It will germinate from seed but follow the instructions on the seed packet *exactly*. It needs some pre-planting preparation.

Calendula: Although Calendula is supposed to be a perennial herb, I've found it best to count on one packet of seeds producing plants for two years. After that, I have to overseed. You'll be able to support three or four plants in a 10 inch pot. Unfortunately, Calendula only produces one flower per plant so you won't have much unless you seed more than one pot.

Catnip: is a member of the Mint family and like all Mints, grows easily and spreads rapidly. Thin to three plants in the pot and allow one to go to seed for more plants next year. If you have cats, I suggest you keep this somewhere they can't get to. Otherwise, they'll have all the fun and you won't have much to harvest. Catnip will also tolerate partial shade.

Comfrey: If you've got a friend that already has Comfrey planted, all you need is the gift of a piece of root. If not, it's easier to get a plant than try to grow it from seed. As you want the roots of 2-year old plants, this cuts down on the time to harvest considerably. You can grow 2 plants per 10 inch pot. When you harvest, break off a piece of root & re-plant for your next crop.

Garlic/Onion: Didn't think of planting these indoors, did you? As long as your pot is at least eight inches deep, you can grow them in pots. For Garlic, you can either buy 'seed stock' over the internet or simply divide a bulb you've purchased at the grocery store down to its individual cloves, and plant them point-end up in your pot, about five inches apart (you can get three in a 10 inch pot). Onions grow easily from seed and you can start them indoors anytime.

Lavender: Also grows, but not so easily, from seed. I've found it easiest to buy plants at the nursery. If you grow from seed, be aware that it will take 2-3 years before you have a plant that produces enough flowers to use.

Lemon/Lime/Orange: Didn't think about these, either? Horticulturalists have come up with dwarf trees that with proper attention will give you lovely fruit inside or on a balcony or patio. These *do* require some close attention at times, and a much larger pot to support a tree. Unless you live in southern climes, you'll want to bring these indoors in the winter.

Mugwort: If you're a witch, you probably want Mugwort around. It grows easily from seed, doesn't require a lot of attention and doesn't mind being a bit crowded in a pot. You can grow up to four plants in a 10 inch pot.

Rose: One plant, one pot, lots of flowers. Buy bare root stock at the nursery, plant it in your pot and *baby* it. This is another plant that is happiest in full sun so if you don't have it, get a grow light.

Rosemary: will grow indoors – with proper attention. Remember that it is a native of the Mediterranean so likes a lot of sun and the *proper* amount of moisture. This plant will die if you overwater it! You won't have to water it as often in the summer but pay close attention to soil moisture in the winter – forced-air heat dries dirt quickly. I've never tried growing it from seed and understand it can be quite difficult. My first plants were purchased from the nursery and subsequent ones were rooted from cuttings. This is another plant that doesn't like winter so be sure to bring it indoors before the first frost.

Sage: Like almost all members of the Mint family, grows easily from seed and spreads rapidly. Be sure you thin your new plants to no more than two in a 10 inch pot. It doesn't share well. Clary Sage grows as easily but unless you live in the desert, I wouldn't recommend you try White Sage, especially indoors. It likes to be drier than is truly healthy for a human.

Thyme: also grows easily from seed, especially *Thymus vulgaris*. One plant, one pot. It will grow into a small bush a foot or more high and wide if you let it.

If you get a *little* sun each day, try:

Angelica: Grows nicely from seed. Ensure your pot is either very wide or very tall as Angelica also grows tall – up to six feet!

Lemon Balm (Melissa): As a member of the Mint family, grows easily and spreads rapidly. However, it's delicate – full sun will burn its leaves. Therefore, partial sun to full shade only.

Oregano: also grows easily from seed. Only one or two plants per pot will provide you enough leaves for a lifetime of Italian cooking. Be sure to pinch it back regularly or it will get rather leggy.

Parsley: does not germinate easily from seed. If you want to try, read the seed packet carefully as it requires some pre-planting preparation. I find it easiest to purchase a plant from the nursery. (An added benefit – you'll have access to a wide variety of Parsleys that aren't always available as seeds.)

Full shade herbs are few & far between, but:

Chamomile: Has delicate, fern-like leaves that *will* grow in full sun but prefers partial- to full-shade. Because of the way it grows, you'll only be able to get one or two plants per pot, which won't yield *a lot* of flowers. If growing indoors, plan on re-seeding every year so you can harvest all your flowers without allowing some to go to seed.

Ginger: really likes a moist, woodland-type environment. Almost full shade with only filtered sunlight works best, here. Rather than try seeds, buy a fresh root at the grocery store, put it somewhere cool for a month or two, then break (don't cut) the root apart & plant the pieces. The fewer plants per pot, the larger your root will grow.

Mints: any mint will grow almost anywhere but you'll find they're happiest in partial- to full-shade. They'll smell stronger, too. If you choose to plant both Peppermint and Spearmint, keep them far apart! Otherwise they will hybridize and you'll end up with a plant that is neither.

This is only a sampling of herbs that can be grown indoors. If there's an herb you really like, chances are you can grow it. A quick Internet search will tell you if it'll like your climate and how to take care of it.

Notes

Appendix A
Preparations

Interestingly enough, many types of herbal preparations are useful in both a medicinal *and* magical context. As you're doing your research, you'll find out which types of preparations work best in a given situation.

In this section I'm going to always use dried herbs unless otherwise noted. Be aware that for the most part, dried herbs are twice as strong as fresh so if you're using fresh, double the amount in your recipe. Also be sure you slightly crush your herbs to open pores and release the plants' oils.

The easiest method to use herbs is in **food**. You have to eat, so why not? You can make a very healthful meal using fruits and vegetables and adding some herbs. Or, you can make your meal a truly magical one by reciting your spell as you're cooking.

The most widely used preparation is a **tea** or tisane. (Actually, Tea is an herb. Its Latin binomial is *Camellia sinensis*.) Medicinally it's called an infusion or decoction. Magically, it's usually called a brew, potion or philter. To make a tea of a leaf or flower (an infusion) put one teaspoon herb in one cup just-boiled water. The water should be still steaming but not bubbling. Cover the cup to prevent the steam from escaping and allow it to steep for about ten minutes. Strain before use or use a tea bag or ball. To make a tea of a root or bark (a decoction), put one teaspoon herb in one and a half cups *cold* water. Bring the water to a boil, reduce the heat and allow it to simmer until your liquid is reduced to one cup. Again, strain before use.

I'm sure you know you can drink the tea (but be sure the herb is safe to ingest, first). A tea is used to make a **fomentation**. Prepare a strong infusion or decoction (double the amount of herb you use) and then soak a cloth in it. Bind the cloth around the area of the body you want to affect and cover with another cloth. This is very useful not only medicinally but in magical health workings targeted to a specific part of the body. You can also use a tea in skin preparations; as a wash, whether for yourself, your house or your magical items; or swish it into your bath water.

A **Poultice** is used in the same way as a fomentation to affect a part of the body. In this case, make a mash of herb(s) and warm water and apply directly to the skin. Cover with a warm cloth. Do not use a poultice if the skin is broken or inflamed. Use a fomentation instead.

Tinctures or **Simples** are an alcoholic extract of a single herb. They are a great way to use herbs medicinally, especially if you're taking or using more than one. A tincture is much more portable than trying to haul all the accoutrements for making tea. In addition, it's a lot easier to get down if the herb tastes bad (and many do). The folk method of making a tincture is to put one ounce herb into one pint good-quality vodka or brandy and let it steep for about 2 weeks, shaking it once a day. If the herb absorbs the liquid (many will), add more vodka or brandy until the level is about one-quarter inch above the herb. Strain well (use a coffee filter to get all the dregs), bottle and store in a cool, dark place. The alcohol acts as a preserving agent and tinctures will last for up to four years. Medicinally, put drops of the tincture (usually fifteen to thirty) into a glass of water or juice to drink, or dilute it further for a skin preparation. Magically, tinctures are used in the same way as a tea and can also charge paper used for written work. Soak the paper in the tincture and let it dry before using.

If you're averse to the use of alcohol in any form, you can make tinctures from apple cider vinegar or vegetable glycerin. Just be aware that your preparation won't be as potent. Also, if you make a vinegar tincture, be sure to use a jar *without* a metal lid. The fumes from the vinegar will corrode the metal.

Herbal Wine is a tasty way of taking your medicine. A cup of wine can be drunk as part of a magical working, too. To make an herbal wine, use the same method as a tincture, substituting either red or white wine for the brandy or vodka (red will be more medicinally-potent). Or, go all-out and make your own wine from virtually any berry.

Pure **Essential Oils** are the best-smelling way to use herbs. They are the "volatile oil" component of a plant and are extracted through a distillation process. They are also *strong* and can be toxic. Lavender, Tea Tree and in some instances, Clove are the only ones you can apply directly on your skin without worrying about overdosing. Never use any other essential oil directly on the skin without first diluting it in a base oil (see infused oils for a partial list). And, *never* ingest an essential oil unless you're under the guidance of a certified aromatherapist. Because they are so strong, it only takes about ten drops to one-eighth cup (one ounce) of base oil. To mix your oils, put the essential oils in the bottle first, then add the base oil. Cap and turn the bottle up and down in your hand ten times before using. Be aware of the difference between an "essential oil" and a "fragrance oil". Fragrance oils are usually synthetic and, if they have any therapeutic actions or magical energies at all, they're not the same ones as true essential oils. Also be aware that there is a difference in qualities of essential oils. The purer the oil, the better. Again, as close to the natural plant as possible. You'll pay for the good stuff but it's worth it. You can use essential oils in your skin care preparations, swish a few drops into your bath or put a few drops into a steam vaporizer and inhale the fumes. Magically, dab the oil onto your pulse points, put a few drops onto a handkerchief to carry with you, rub it into candles or burn it in an oil warmer or on charcoal. If you choose to burn the oil on charcoal, be aware that the aroma won't last longer than a few seconds. Again, if you're going to come into skin contact, be sure to dilute the essential oil first. Essential oils will keep for two to five years. As a general rule, the thicker the oil, the longer it will keep. Be sure to keep the bottle tightly capped as air will destroy the oil faster.

Hydrosols or **Flower Waters** are a by-product when essential oils are obtained by a steam distillation method. Even though they are known as "flower waters", a hydrosol is simply a distillation of any part of the plant that contains essential oils, like the leaves or inner bark. You can buy them commercially or, with a little effort, make your own. Small commercial stills are available so you can make your own essential oils and hydrosols. If you don't want to buy a still, you can get almost the same effect on your stove. You'll want a large (20 quart or so) pot that has a domed lid. Put about three quarts of water and ten ounces of *fresh* herb in the pot and let it sit for a few hours before proceeding. Then put a vegetable steamer basket upside down in the center of the pot and a cereal-sized bowl right-side up on top of the basket to catch the hydrosol. Cover and bring to just under a boil. As soon as the water begins to simmer, reduce the heat, turn the lid upside down on the pot and put a large bag of ice in the lid. The ice will help condense the steam faster. The hydrosol is the condensed steam that will drip from the lid into your cereal bowl. Be sure to keep an eye on your preparation – make sure the water doesn't boil away and burn your herb. Once you've obtained a goodly amount of hydrosol in your cereal bowl, remove everything from the heat and allow to cool. Pour the water from the bowl through a coffee filter into a sterile bottle, then refrigerate. If you're lucky, you'll also have a few drops of essential oil in the bottom of the filter. Draw this off with a pipette and put into a separate bottle.

If you don't want to go to the trouble of distilling, you can pour two cups of boiling water over one cup of tightly-packed, fresh herb. Allow your mixture to cool completely, strain and pour into a sterilized bottle. This will not be as strong-smelling as a distilled hydrosol but is a simpler method.

An even quicker method of making a flower water involves essential oils. To one-quarter cup of distilled water, add six to eight drops of your chosen essential oil and bottle. Shake before use. This will have a much lighter fragrance than a regular hydrosol and is known as a "voile", which is French for "veil".

Hydrosols are generally used for skin issues, most often as an ingredient in a cream. However, Rose water on its own is an ages-old natural skin cleanser and astringent. My grandmother used to sprinkle her bedsheets with Lavender water. This not only kept bugs out of the bed but they smelled wonderful. Magically you can use them for asperging, sprinkling or virtually anywhere you would use a tea or brew.

The use of **Ointments** is pretty much limited to the skin. (I'm not sure why you would want to eat an ointment!) Medicinally, rub them into the area you want to affect, like a sore muscle or on a rash. Magically, massage it into pulse points to get the energies into your body. The old method of making an ointment was to use lard but nowadays, vegetable shortening is available and smells *much* better. Melt one cup shortening over low heat (do not allow it to get so hot the shortening smokes). Add three tablespoons of dried herb(s) and allow to "cook" for about ten minutes. Strain and cool the mixture before use. Or, melt the shortening and add up to ten drops of essential oils before cooling. If you like something firmer than shortening, add a couple of tablespoons of melted beeswax to the mixture. You can also use anhydrous lanolin (available in health food stores) with a little beeswax to thicken the mixture. A caution: if you're allergic to wool, don't use lanolin. It's the oil collected from the skin of sheep, which is where wool comes from, too. Ointments should be stored in an airtight container in a cool, dark place.

Infused Oils can be used the same as an ointment, as an all-over massage oil or as a salad dressing. There are a variety of good base oils on the market today but the easiest is plain ol' cold-pressed, extra virgin olive oil, which is available on virtually every grocer's shelf. My personal feeling is that olive oil is a bit too heavy to use for most skin preparations and it does have a distinct smell so other, lighter options include apricot, avocado, cocoanut, grapeseed, and sweet almond. (If ordering cocoanut oil over the Internet, be sure to get the "fractionated" kind. Cocoanut oil is solid in its normal state.) Jojoba oil is also available but it's actually a liquid wax and is somewhat heavy. It is also more expensive compared to other alternatives. Put one part herb in ten parts oil (the equivalent of one ounce by weight of herb in ten fluid ounces oil) into a jar that has a tight-fitting lid. Place in a cool, dark place. Shake ten times once a day for ten days. Strain, bottle and store in a cool, dark place. If you want a stronger infused oil, simply strain out the herb and repeat the process. Use your original oil and add another batch of herbs in the same proportion as the first time. With the exception of jojoba oil, all oils have a shelf life, which varies by oil. Be sure to make only small batches and store unused portions in the refrigerator to keep your oils fresher longer.

Incense of the "raw" or "granular" type is just plant material smoldered on a charcoal tablet. The use of incense has been documented for over 5,000 years. Although today "fumigation" generally means "pest control", it really means "to apply smoke". Even after World War I, French hospitals not only strewed herbs on the floor, they wafted the smoke of burning herbs in the sick wards to purify the air. Incense smoke can be used to purify the air in a room; its vibrations are great as background when you're meditating; or you can pass ritual items through the smoke to purify them. Pick an herb or combination thereof and grind it down to about the size of peppercorns or coarsely-ground salt. Light the edge of a charcoal tablet held in a heat-proof container and once the tablet is fully lit, sprinkle a small amount of your herb onto the tablet every few minutes. Easy does it! You don't want to set off your smoke alarm. Also remember that a lot of herbs don't smell as good while burning as you might think.

If you've a mind, you can make your own cone or stick incense: choose your herbs, add a little gum arabic or gum traganth (to make it sticky), and either charcoal or saltpeter (for combustion). Powder your ingredients very, very fine. Mix your powder with a little distilled water to make a dough and then form into cones or roll around bamboo sticks. Place on a sheet of waxed paper and allow to dry at least two or three weeks, turning every couple of days to expose all surfaces to air. I haven't included any proportions because the recipe varies depending on the herbs used and your climate. You'll need to experiment on your own and be sure to keep a record!

Baths, believe it or not, do have a medicinal application. They are great to loosen tense muscles, for some skin issues, and for problems in the genital area. They are a luxurious method of herbal magic – especially if you add some soap to make a bubble bath. This spreads the herb's energies all over your body. You can use a tea, essential oils or bath salts in your bath.

To make bath salts, add up to fifteen drops of essential oil(s) into one cup Epsom salts or a combination of sea and Epsom salts – add until your nose tells you its right. (You can also use rock salt but you'll probably have to grind it down a bit as it's usually sold in largish chunks.) It's easiest to make your salts in a jar with a lid. This way you can shake to mix. I prefer to mix them in a bowl and use my hands to get *my* energies into the salts. If you want to color your salts, use food coloring and definitely use the shaker-jar method. It will only take a few drops to completely color a cup of salts. (If you overdo it on the food coloring, you will color yourself and your tub. Therefore, if you want a darker color, use either food-grade dyes or dyes specifically made for soaps.) Again, mix thoroughly to disperse the coloring throughout. Put two to four tablespoons of your salt mixture into a warm bath and swish around a bit. Only soak for about ten minutes if you're using salts. You'll re-absorb all the toxins your body has released into the bath if you soak longer.

If you don't like to take baths (or don't have a bathtub) you can get the same effect in the shower by using finer-ground salts as a body scrub or putting herbs in a sachet bag and hanging it from the showerhead so the water flows through the bag and then onto you.

I wouldn't recommend that you use loose herbs in either the bath or shower. They have a tendency to clog up the pipes and that sort of problem generates negative thoughts and energy, as well as high plumber's bills. Instead, either brew a tea and put that into your bathwater or as noted before, put the loose herbs in a sachet bag and allow the water to run through the bag. If you're in a romantic mood, by all means float a few rose petals on the surface of your bath but be sure to scoop them out before pulling the plug.

Soaps are another way to use herbs in the bath or shower, either medicinally or magically. They have become popular as a craft in recent years and soap-making kits are readily available at craft stores. You can powder dried herbs and add these to your mixture (ground oatmeal is great as a skin softener) or add a few drops of essential oil.

Sachets or herbal **Amulets** are an easy way to carry an herb (or a combination of herbs) with you all day long. I've seen sachets used as decongestants: they contain strong-smelling herbs such as Eucalyptus. One inhales the aroma to clear up congestion. For magical purposes you can carry a piece of dried herb in your pocket (like carrying a "lucky" Buckeye) or follow the example of the residents of the Isle of Man: on Tynwald Day (St. John's Feast Day), everyone wears a sprig of Mugwort in their lapel. Although Mugwort is the Manx official flower, this is a holdover from the Middle Ages when wearing a crown or carrying a posy of Mugwort was thought to ward off witchcraft. (Little did they know that most witches consider Mugwort one of their favorite herbs!)

A small muslin bag that has a drawstring or a small piece of cotton cloth that has been sewn up works great to carry a combination of herbs (or you can simply place the herb in the middle of a square of cloth, pull the corners together and use a ribbon to tie it up).

Select the herb(s) you want to use, put a small amount in the bag and close it. Carry it in your pocket or somewhere on your person so the herbs can add their energies to yours during the day. Sachets can also be hung over doors or beds, in cars or placed wherever they can do the most good. Remember to replace your sachet every three months and recycle (compost) the herbs back to the Earth.

Pillows are usually used for dream magic or nightly protection but can be made for any type of magic. They should be fairly small (no more than 6" x 6"). Use those small squares of fabric you bought to make your sachets. Take two pieces, stitch up three sides and fill before closing the fourth side. You can fill them with dried herbs and add other things germane to your work like gems or other objects (you don't actually have to sleep *on* them, just have them near you at night). Aromatherapy has heightened the interest in dream pillows. A dream pillow made of sedative herbs can be used for insomnia. You can make your pillow stronger-smelling by putting a few drops of essential oils onto the dried herbs. Again, recycle the herbs every three months or so.

Powders are simply finely ground herbs. Sprinkle powders around your house or area where you're performing your magic or use them as incense. Yarrow (*Achillea millefolium*) powder is a good styptic (to staunch bleeding). A medicinal note: one-third teaspoon powder is equal to two 00 capsules.

Candles can also be used with herbs! If you make your own candles, you can powder herbs and add them to the hot wax or add a few drops of essential oil(s) prior to pouring into your chosen mold or container. If you use store-bought candles, 'dress' them by rubbing a little vegetable oil on the candle and then roll it lightly in powdered herbs. Don't use too much of your herbal powder as it tends to burn quickly and can cause a flash fire similar to sawdust.

You can also put a drop or two of essential oil into the puddle of wax formed around a burning wick.

Pomanders are what I made as a kid at Christmas. Mom hung them up in the house; they looked pretty and made the house smell good. However, they do have a magical application. Depending on what you're trying to accomplish, you'll stud a citrus fruit with cloves, roll it in other powdered herbs, tie it with a ribbon and hang it up in your house. Not only will the house smell good but you'll be infusing the area with magical intentions. These will need to be recycled every few weeks as the fruit won't last as long as the herbs.

Poppets are generally associated with negative magic but they do have a positive use, especially for healing, love, and fertility spells. You can make one out of wax, clay or papier mâché; or simply use a child's doll that you have altered to look as much like the person in question as possible. If you make one from scratch, be sure to leave a hollow area – usually in the torso but sometimes in the head. You can stuff the poppet with herbs appropriate to the situation or if you need to do a health working for a specific part of the body, the poppet makes a good substitute for the sore leg or broken arm you need to heal that is 100 miles away. Apply a poultice or fomentation to the area on the poppet corresponding to the body part that needs healing.

Magical Inks are used when a spell requires something written. Many practitioners use magical inks when writing in their Workbook. They are sometimes made with resins (most often Dragon's Blood which is red, unlike most other resins which are clear to whitish), lampblack (very tedious), or you can simply crush fresh fruit (like elderberries) and use the juice as an "ink". You'll want a pen you can use with your ink – a fountain, feather or wood pen that can either draw the ink into its own well or be used dipping-style. If you've never used a dipping pen, be sure to practice with it before writing in your Workbook or using it for a written working. Practice until you're proficient enough to write without smears and blotches.

If you want to go all the way and make your own ink, here's how you make ink with lampblack. Light a candle of a color appropriate to your intention. (This was once done with oil lamps instead of candles, hence the name "lampblack".) Once the flame takes hold, hold a spoon over the flame. You'll soon see soot starting to collect on the spoon. As you get a good coating, use a knife to scrape the soot into a bowl. Repeat. And repeat. It's not only very time-consuming, it's also very messy as the flakes won't always cooperate and float directly into your bowl. Once you've collected enough soot flakes, add distilled water until your mixture is thin enough to use. You can use the same method but instead of using a candle, use the soot of burning resin(s) like Frankincense or Myrrh.

To make an ink with Dragon's Blood, soak a tablespoon of crushed resin in five tablespoons of alcohol (grain alcohol is best but 90 proof vodka will work). It will take an hour or so, but when the two substances have combined well, you'll have a very red liquid substance in your bowl. Strain out any remaining resin. Add some powdered gum arabic or gum traganth to thicken enough for use.

You can also use charcoal as an ink. Simply take a dried twig of an appropriate tree, light the end, gently blow the flame out and allow it to smolder until the end is blackened enough to write with. Be sure to wait until it stops smoldering before actually writing on paper or you may have a conflagration on your hands. You'll have to pause and relight often to keep the end black.

However, there is an easier method to make (and use) magical ink. You can magically charge a bottle of regular ink by adding essential oils and your own energies to one you've purchased. I generally add fifteen drops to a one ounce bottle of ink. Any more and the ink gets too oily to adhere to paper.

Paper can be magically charged for written work ... either your Workbook or a written spell. I have read that parchment paper should be used because "its organic properties are compatible with nature". Parchment is traditionally made from calfskin, goatskin or sheepskin; there are still sources out there for this type and I'm sure that it's all ethically made. However, it's *expensive*, so I use plant-based parchment – writing paper! If you choose to use magical ink with a dipping-style pen, I believe you'll find that using a heavier grade of paper than simply notebook or copier paper will work better – the ink won't bleed through to the other side as easily. There are plenty of heavier-weight papers available at office supply stores that will suffice. To charge paper, soak it in a tincture or put a few drops of essential oil(s) onto the page (use herbs associated with your project) and let it air dry.

If you're really into crafts and the "do-it-all-yourself" mentality, you can make your own paper. I haven't tried but there are quite a few books and web sites that give good instructions for doing so. Again, use herbs appropriate to your project.

Washes can be used to cleanse the solid surfaces in your house or as sprinkling (asperging) waters. To a cup of distilled water (always used distilled to avoid any unpleasant additions from tap water), add up to fifteen drops of your chosen essential oils. Or, make an infusion or decoction with dried herbs but again, use the distilled water. If you're going to clean anyways, combine one tablespoon of dish soap with your cup of distilled water mixture. Then add that to your bucket of cleaning water.

Appendix B
Herbal Cheat Sheet

Throughout this book I've used the Common Names by which I know the herbs. This list will help you identify the *exact* herb I'm referring to.

Common Name	Latin Binomial
Agrimony	*Agrimonia eupatoria*
Alfalfa	*Medicago Sativa*
Allspice	*Pimenta dioica*
Aloe Vera	*Aloe barbadensis*
Angelica	*Angelica archangelica*
Anise	*Pimpinella anisum*
Apple	*Pyrus malus*
Arnica	*Arnica montana*
Asafoetida	*Ferula assa-foetida*
Ashwagandha	*Withania somnifera*
Aspen	*Populus spp.*
Astragalus	*Astragalus spp.*
Barberry	*Berberis vulgaris*
Barley	*Hordeum distichon*
Basil (Sweet)	*Ocimum basilicum*
Bay	*Laurus nobilis*
Bayberry	*Myrica cerifera*

Beet (White or Red)	*Beta vulgaris*
Benzoin	*Styrax benzoin*
Bergamot	*Citrus bergamia*
Bilberry	*Vaccinium myrtillus*
Bindweed	*Convolvulus sepium*
Birch	*Betula alba*
Bistort	*Polygonum bistorta*
Black Cohosh	*Cimicifuga racemosa*
Black Haw	*Viburnum prunifolium*
Blackberry	*Rubus villosus*
Bladderwrack	*Fucus vesiculosus*
Blessed Thistle	*Cnicus benedictus*
Bloodroot	*Sanguinaria canadensis*
Blue Flag	*Iris versicolor*
Blueberry	*Vaccinium myrtillus*
Boneset	*Eupatorium perfoliatum*
Broom	*Cytisus scoparius*
Bryonia	*Bryonia spp.*
Buckthorn	*Rhamnus frangula*
Buckwheat	*Fagopyrum esculentum*
Burdock	*Arctium lappa*
Cabbage	*Brassica oleracea*
Cajeput	*Melaleuca leucadendron*
Calendula	*Calendula officinalis*
Camphor	*Cinnamomum camphora*
Caraway	*Carum carvi*
Cardamom	*Eletteria cardamomum*
Cascara Sagrada	*Rhamnus purshiana*
Catnip	*Nepeta cataria*
Cayenne	*Capsicum minimum*

Cedar	*Cedrus spp.*
Celandine	*Chelidonium majus*
Celery	*Apium graveolens*
Centaury	*Erythraea centarium*
Chamomile, German	*Matricaria recutita*
Chamomile, Roman	*Chamamelum nobile*
Chasteberry	*Vitex agnus-castus*
Cherry, Black	*Prunus serotina*
Cherry, Sweet	*Prunus avium*
Cherry, Wild	*Prunus serotina*
Chestnut	*Castanea sativa*
Chestnut, Horse	*Aesculus hippocastanum*
Chickweed	*Stellaria media*
Chives	*Allium schoenoprasum*
Cinnamon	*Cinnamomum cassia*
Cleavers	*Galium aparine*
Clover (Red)	*Trifolium pratense*
Cloves	*Syzgium aromaticum*
Coconut	*Cocos nucifera*
Coffee	*Coffea spp.*
Coltsfoot	*Tussilago farfara*
Comfrey	*Symphytum officinale*
Copal	*Bursera fagaroides*
Corn	*Zea mays*
Crampbark	*Viburnum opulus*
Cranberry	*Vaccinum erythrocarpum*
Cucumber	*Cucumis sativus*
Cumin	*Cuminum cyminum*
Cypress	*Cupressus sempervirens*
Dandelion	*Taraxacum officinale*

Deer's Tongue	*Trilisa odoratissima*
Dill	*Anethum graveolens*
Dragon's Blood	*Daemonorops draco*
Echinacea	*Echinacea spp.*
Elder (Black)	*Sambucus nigra*
Elecampane	*Inula helenium*
Elm, Slippery	*Ulmus fulva*
Endive	*Cichorium endivia*
Eucalyptus	*Eucalyptus globulus*
Evening Primrose	*Oenothera spp.*
Eyebright	*Euphrasia officinalis*
Fennel	*Foeniculum vulgare*
Fenugreek	*Trigonella foenum-graecum*
Feverfew	*Tanacetum parthenium*
Flax	*Linim usitatissimum*
Frankincense	*Boswellia carterii*
Galangal	*Alpinia officinarum*
Gardenia	*Gardenia jasminoides*
Garlic	*Allium sativum*
Gelsemium	*Gelsemium sempervirens*
Gentian	*Gentiana lutea*
Geranium	*Pelargonium spp.*
Ginger	*Zingiber officinale*
Gingko	*Gingko biloba*
Ginseng, American	*Panax quinquefolius*
Ginseng, Siberian	*Eleutherococcus senticosus*
Goldenseal	*Hydrastis canadensis*
Gooseberry	*Ribes spp.*
Gotu Kola	*Centella asiatica*
Grape	*Vitis vinifera*

Gravel Root	*Eupatorium purpureum*
Hawthorn	*Crataegus laevigata*
Hazel	*Corylus spp.*
Hibiscus	*Hibiscus sabdariffa*
High John the Conqueror	*Ipomoea purga*
Holly	*Ilex aquifolium*
Hollyhock	*Althea rosea*
Honeysuckle	*Lonicera caprifolium*
Hops	*Humulus lupulus*
Horehound (White)	*Marrubium vulgare*
Horse Chestnut	*Aesculus hippocastanum*
Horseradish	*Armoracia rusticana*
Hyacinth	*Hyacinthus orientalis*
Hyssop	*Hyssopus officinalis*
Iceland Moss	*Centraria islandica*
Irish Moss	*Chondrus crispus*
Jasmine	*Jasminum officinale*
Joe Pye Weed	*Eupatorium purpureum*
Juniper	*Juniperus communis*
Kelp	*Fucus vesiculosus*
Lady's Mantle	*Alchemilla vulgaris*
Lavender	*Lavandula angustifolia*
Lemon	*Citrus limon*
Lemon Balm	*Melissa officinalis*
Lemongrass	*Cymbopogon citratus*
Licorice	*Glycyrrhiza glabra*
Linden	*Tilia platyphyllos*
Lobelia	*Lobelia inflata*
Lovage	*Levisticum officinale*
Mandrake	*Mandragora officinarum*

Marjoram	*Origanum vulgare*
Marshmallow	*Althaea officinalis*
Meadowsweet	*Filipendula ulmaria*
Milk Thistle	*Silybum marianum*
Mistletoe	*Viscum album*
Motherwort	*Leonurus cardiaca*
Mugwort	*Artemisia vulgaris*
Mullein	*Verbascum thapsus*
Mustard (Black)	*Brassica nigra*
Myrrh	*Commiphora molmol*
Nettle	*Urtica dioica*
Nutmeg	*Myristica fragrans*
Oak	*Quercus alba*
Oat	*Avena sativa*
Oatstraw	*Avena sativa*
Onion	*Allium cepa*
Orange (Sweet)	*Citrus sinensis*
Orchid	*Orchis spp.*
Oregano	*Origanum vulgare*
Oregon Grape	*Mahonia aquifolium*
Orris	*Iris germanica var. florentina*
Palmarosa	*Cymbopogon martinii*
Pansy	*Viola tricolor*
Parsley	*Petroselinum crispum*
Passionflower	*Passiflora incarnata*
Patchouli	*Pogostemon cablin*
Pecan	*Carya illinoinensis*
Pepper (Black)	*Piper nigrum*
Peppermint	*Mentha x piperita*
Petitgrain	*Citrus aurantium var. amara*

Pine	*Pinus spp.*
Pineapple	*Ananas comosus*
Plantain (Broad-leafed)	*Plantago major*
Poke	*Phytolacca americana*
Pomegranate	*Punica granatum*
Poppy	*Papaver spp.*
Primrose	*Primula vulgaris*
Primrose, Evening	*Oenothera spp.*
Pumpkin	*Cucurbita pepo*
Raspberry (Red)	*Rubus idaeus*
Red Clover	*Trifolium pratense*
Rhubarb, Turkey	*Rheum officinale*
Rice	*Oryza sativa*
Rose	*Rosa spp.*
Rosemary	*Rosmarinus officinalis*
Rue	*Ruta graveolens*
Sage	*Salvia officinalis*
Sage, Clary	*Salvia sclarea*
Sage, White	*Salvia apiana*
Sandalwood (Red)	*Pterocarpus santalinus*
Sandalwood (White)	*Santalum album*
Savory	*Satureja hortensis*
Saw Palmetto	*Serenoa repens*
Scullcap	*Scutellaria lateriflora*
Sea Holly	*Eryngium spp.*
Senna	*Senna alexandrina*
Skunk Cabbage	*Symplocarpus foetidus*
Slippery Elm	*Ulmus fulva*
Spearmint	*Mentha spicata*
St. John's Wort	*Hypericum perforatum*

Stevia	*Stevia rebaudiana*
Strawberry	*Fragaria vesca*
Sunflower	*Helianthus annuus*
Sweet Grass	*Hierochloe odorata*
Tea	*Camellia sinensis*
Tea Tree	*Melaleuca alternifolia*
Thyme	*Thymus vulgaris*
Turkey Rhubarb	*Rheum officinale*
Turmeric	*Curcuma longa*
Uva Ursi	*Arctostaphylos uva-ursi*
Valerian	*Valeriana officinalis*
Vanilla	*Vanilla spp.*
Vervain	*Verbena officinalis*
Vetivert	*Chrysopogon zizinoides*
Violet, Sweet	*Viola odorata*
Vitex	*Vitex agnus-castus*
Walnut (Black)	*Juglans nigra*
Watercress	*Nasturtium officinale*
Watermelon	*Citrus lanatus*
Willow (White)	*Salix alba*
Witch Hazel	*Hamamelis virginiana*
Wood Betony	*Stachys officinalis*
Wormwood	*Artemisia absinthium*
Yarrow	*Achillea millefolium*
Yellow Dock	*Rumex crispus*
Ylang Ylang	*Canaga odorata*
Yucca	*Yucca spp.*

Appendix C
Herbal Therapeutic Actions

Term	Definition
Adaptogen	An herb that increases the body's resistance to stress, trauma, anxiety and fatigue.
Adjuvant	A substance that aids another, such as an auxiliary remedy; a nonspecific stimulator of the immune response.
Alterative	An herb that gradually cleanses the blood by regulating the eliminative organs.
Anodyne	Herbs used to allay pain – usually used when speaking about external treatments.
Analgesic	Herbs used to allay pain when administered orally.
Anthelmintic	Herbs that destroy worms
Antibacterial	Herbs that destroy bacteria or suppress their growth or multiplication
Antibiotic	Herbs that have the capacity to inhibit the growth of or to kill other microorganisms.
Antiemetic	Herbs that prevent or alleviate nausea or vomiting.

Antimicrobial	Herbs that will kill microorganisms or suppress their multiplication or growth.
Antioxidant	Herbs that prevent oxidation of other molecules, preventing or delaying deterioration when exposed to air.
Antipyretic	Herbs that reduce fever; see febrifuge.
Antispasmodic	Herbs used to relieve nervous irritability and reduce or prevent excessive involuntary muscular contractions or spasms.
Antiseptic	Herbs used to prevent, resist, and counteract putrefaction (decay of cells and formation of pus).
Antitussive	Prevents coughing.
Antiviral	Herbs that destroy viruses or suppress their growth or multiplication.
Astringent	Herbs that contract tissues make them denser and firmer, slowing down discharges.
Bitter	Herbs that increase the tone of gastrointestinal tissues.
Carminative	Herbs that expel gas from the stomach and intestines.
Decongestant	An herb that reduces congestion in the respiratory tract.
Demulcent	Herbs having mucilaginous properties that are soothing and protective internally to irritated and inflamed surfaces and tissue.

Diaphoretic	Herbs that produce perspiration and increased elimination through the skin.
Diuretic	Herbs that increase the secretion and flow of urine.
Emetic	Herbs that cause vomiting.
Emmenagogue	Herbs that promote menstruation, or restore proper menstrual function.
Emollient	An herb used to soothe and soften the skin (an external demulcent).
Expectorant	An herb that promotes the removal of mucus from the bronchial tubes.
Febrifuge	An herb that reduces fever
Irritant	An herb that irritates tissue, drawing blood to the area that promotes healing.
Laxative	An herb that loosens the bowels and relieves constipation.
Nervine	Herbs that reduce excitement – calming.
Rubefacient	An herb that stimulates circulation and reddens the skin.
Sedative	Herbs that allay irritability and excitement or lessen higher brain functions.
Sialagogue	A drug or other agent that increases the flow of saliva.
Stimulant	An herb that increases activity in the body or in a specific organ.

Tonic	An herb that invigorates and tones up the system.
Vermicide	An herb that kills intestinal worms.
Vermifuge	An herb that expels intestinal worms.
Vulnerary	Herbs that promote healing of wounds.

Appendix D
Measurements & Equivalents

Measure	Equivalent
1 teaspoon (t)	5 mL
1 tablespoon (T)	15 mL
1 ounce (oz)	30 mL
1 cup (C)	8 fluid ounces (fl oz)
1 pint (pt)	16 fl oz
1 quart (qt)	32 fl oz
1 milliliter (mL)	15 drops
1 gram (gm)	.0002 pounds (lb)
1 ounce (oz) dry weight	30 gm

www.ingramcontent.com/pod-product-compliance
Lightning Source LLC
Chambersburg PA
CBHW030013290326

41934CB00005B/323